AF820759

Cells Tissues Organs

in vivo, in vitro

Founded 1945 as 'Acta Anatomica' by R. Chambers, G. Glimstedt, T. Peterfi and G. Wolf-Heidegger
Continued 1962–1974 by E.A. Boyden, 1955–1980 by A. Delmas, 1972–1980 by F. Walberg, 1945–1980 by G. Wolf-Heidegger, 1981–1988 by R. O'Rahilly, Davis, Calif., 1989–1990 by G.E. Goslow, Jr., Providence, R.I., 1981–1992 by W. Lierse, Hamburg

KARGER

Printed in Switzerland on acid-free paper by Reinhardt Druck, Basel

Appears 6-weekly: 2 volumes per year (8 issues)

Guidelines for Authors

Cells Tissues Organs

Aims and Scope

Cells Tissues Organs is an international forum for communication among scientists interested in current research on functional morphology and morphogenesis at all levels of organization, from subcellular to macroscopy, with emphasis on humans and higher vertebrates. The journal offers rapid exchange of novel and significant information gained from experimental and theoretical investigations on all aspects that are pertinent to the formation and transformation of biological structure.

Topics of special interest include

Developmental and reproductive biology, cell biology, tissue engineering, artificial organs, in vitro systems and transplantation. Papers highlighting the links between structural and functional aspects are preferred.

Types of Papers

The journal publishes: (1) Original papers on experimental research. (2) Theoretical contributions. These will appear in the section 'Hypotheses and Concepts' and may include provocative hypotheses, provided that they are innovative, well founded and show promise for new avenues of research. (3) Short reviews/perspectives. While (1) and (2) are submitted contributions, reviews/perspectives (3) are invited. Suggestions concerning reviews on current topics of high interest are welcome.

All manuscripts must be accompanied by a cover letter signed by all authors. Assurance should be given that the manuscript is not under simultaneous consideration by any other publication. Reported studies using animal and human subjects must have been approved by the appropriate institutional review boards.

Submission

Manuscripts from North and South America should be sent to:

Prof. A.W. English, PhD
Emory University School of Medicine
Dept. of Anatomy and Cell Biology
Atlanta, GA 30322 (USA)
Fax +1 404 727–3677
E-Mail cto@cellbio.emory.edu

Manuscripts from Japan and South-East Asia to:

Prof. Dr. Osamu Ohtani
Department of Anatomy II
Toyama Medical and Pharmaceutical University
2630 Sugitani
Toyama, 930-01 (Japan)
Fax +81 764 34 5010

Manuscripts from all other countries to:

Prof. H.-W. Denker
S. Karger AG
Editorial Office 'Cells Tissues Organs'
PO Box
CH–4009 Basel (Switzerland)
Tel. +41 61 306 13 57
Fax +41 61 306 14 34
E-Mail l. haas@karger.ch

Mailing address for courier deliveries only:
Allschwilerstr. 10
CH–4055 Basel (Switzerland)

All manuscripts are subject to peer review. Submission of an article for publication implies the transfer of the copyright from the author to the publisher upon acceptance. Accepted papers become the permanent property of Cells Tissues Organs and may not be reproduced by any means, in whole or in part, without the written consent of the publisher. It is the author's responsibility to obtain permission to reproduce illustrations, tables, etc. from other publications.

Format and Arrangement

Manuscripts should be written in English and be as concise as possible. They should be submitted in quadruplicate (with four sets of original illustrations), typewritten double-spaced on one side of the paper, with a wide margin. *Lines should be numbered in the margin.*

Title page: Title, the authors' names, and the institute where the work was conducted, a short title for use as running head, the full address of the author to whom correspondence should be sent. Please also supply phone and fax numbers, as well as your e-mail address. If different, indicate in addition a full address for revisions and proof reading separately.

Key words: For indexing purposes provide a list of up to 5 key words.

Abstract: Each paper needs an abstract of up to about 20 lines summarizing the essential new information communicated.

Subheadings: Introduction; Materials and Methods; Results; Discussion.

Small type: Paragraphs which can or must be set in smaller type (methods, etc.) should be indicated with a 'p' (petit) in the margin on the left-hand side.

List of Abbreviations: Provide a list of the abbreviations used in your paper. Please list them on a separate page of the manuscript. The list will be printed as a footnote at the bottom of the first page of your article.

Footnotes: With the exception of the list of abbreviations, footnotes should be avoided. When essential, they are numbered consecutively and typed at the foot of the appropriate page.

Nomenclature: The nomenclature used should conform, wherever possible, to the current edition of the Nomina Anatomica (Terminologia Anatomica), Nomina Anatomica Veterinaria, or to the Nomina Anatomica Avium.

Tables and illustrations: Tables and illustrations (both numbered in Arabic numerals) should be prepared on separate sheets. Tables require a heading and figures a legend, also prepared on a separate sheet. For the reproduction of illustrations, only good drawings and original photographs can be accepted; negatives or photocopies cannot be used. Due to technical reasons, figures with a screen background should not be submitted. When possible, group several illustrations on one block for reproduction (max. size 181 × 223 mm) or provide crop marks. On the back of each illustration, indicate its number, the author's name, and 'top' with a soft pencil.

Color illustrations: During the review process, the decision will be made as to which color illustrations of a manuscript can be reproduced free of charge. Authors will be informed of this at the time of acceptance of their paper. Otherwise, these illustrations will be reproduced at the author's expense. Up to 6 color illustrations per page can be integrated into the text at the reduced price of CHF 660.– / USD 545.00 per page.

References: References in the text should be made by author's name followed by the year of publication, arranged chronologically, then alphabetically. When there are more than two authors, use the first author's name and et al. When references are made to more than one paper by the same author, published in the same year, designate them as a, b, c, etc. The list of references should include only those publications which are cited in the text. Material submitted for publication but not yet accepted may be cited in the text as 'unpublished data' but must not be included in the reference list. In the list of references, arrange references alphabetically listing all authors, then year of publication. Abbreviate journal names according to Index Medicus.

Examples

(a) Papers published in periodicals: Sun, J., H. Koto, K.F. Chung (1997) Interaction of ozone and allergen challenges on bronchial responsiveness and inflammation in sensitised guinea pigs. Int Arch Allergy Immunol *112:* 191–195.

Hadler, W.A., S.R. Silveira (1981) Técnica histoquímica que permite discriminar o colesterol de substâncias afins e de seus ésteres. Cienc Cult *33(suppl):* 586–587.

(b) Monographs: Matthews, D.E., V.T. Farewell (1996) Using and Understanding Medical Statistics, ed 3, revised. Basel Karger.

(c) Edited books: Parren, P.W.H.I., D.R. Burton (1997) Antibodies against HIV-1 from phage display libraries: Mapping of an immune response and progress towards antiviral immunotherapy; in Capra, J.D. (ed): Antibody Engineering. Chem Immunol. Basel, Karger, vol 65, pp 18–56.

Further details: Authors may consult the 'Guide to Writing Articles in English' by R. O'Rahilly (Acta Anat *131*: 1–2, 1988).

Galley proofs

Unless indicated otherwise, galley proofs are sent to the first-named author and should be returned with the least possible delay. Alterations made in proofs, other than the correction of printer's errors, are charged to the author.

Reprints

Order forms and a price list are sent with the proofs. Orders submitted after the issue is printed are subject to considerably higher prices.

KARGER

Fax+ 41 61 306 12 34
E-Mail karger@karger.ch
www.karger.com

The Guidelines for Authors are available at:
www.karger.com/journals/cto/cto_gl.htm

General Information

Cells Tissues Organs

Publication data: 'Cells Tissues Organs' is published 8 times a year. Volumes 168–169 with 4 issues each appear in 2001.

Subscription rates: Subscriptions run for a full calendar year. Prices are given per volume.
Personal subscription:
Subscription + postage and handling
CHF 97.– + CHF 18.25 Europe
CHF 97.– + CHF 27.20 Overseas
USD 74.00 + USD 18.25
+ online subscription per volume:
CHF 39.– / USD 30.00
(Must be in the name of, billed to, and paid by an individual. Order must be marked 'personal subscription'.)
Institutional subscription:
Subscription + postage and handling
CHF 927.– + CHF 22.80 Europe
CHF 927.– + CHF 34.– Overseas
USD 713.00 + USD 22.80
+ online subscription per volume:
CHF 58.– / USD 45.00
Airmail postage: CHF 24.–, USD 20.00.
(Extra per volume.)

Microforms: Please direct all enquiries and orders to: University Microfilms Inc.
300 North Zeeb Road, P.O. Box 1346
Ann Arbor, MI 48106-1346 (USA)

Subscription orders: Orders can be placed at agencies, bookstores, directly with the Publisher
S. Karger AG, P.O. Box,
CH–4009 Basel (Switzerland)
or with any of the following distributors:
Deutschland: S. Karger GmbH, Postfach
D–79095 Freiburg
France: Librairie Luginbühl
36, bd de Latour-Maubourg, F–75007 Paris
Great Britain, Ireland: S. Karger Publishers
58 Grove Hill Road
Tunbridge Wells, Kent TN1 1SP, UK
USA: S. Karger Publishers, Inc.
26 West Avon Road, P.O. Box 529
Farmington, CT 06085, USA
India, Bangladesh, Sri Lanka:
Panther Publishers Private Ltd.
39, 6th Cross
Wilson Gardens
Bangalore 560 027, India
Japan: Katakura Libri, Inc.
2F, Marushima Bldg, 4-6-17, Yushima,
Bunkyo-ku, Tokyo 113-0034, Japan

Change of address: Both old and new address should be sent to the subscription source.

Single issues and back volumes: Information can be obtained through the Publisher.

Advertising: Correspondence and rate requests should be addressed to the Publisher.

Bibliographic indices: This journal is regularly listed in bibliographic services, including *Current Contents®*.

Copying: This journal has been registered with the Copyright Clearance Center (CCC), as indicated by the code appearing on the first page of each article.
For readers in the US, this code signals consent for copying of articles for personal or internal use, or for the personal or internal use of specific clients, provided that the stated fee is paid per copy directly to
Copyright Clearance Center Inc.
222 Rosewood Drive
Danvers, MA 01923 (USA)
A copy of the first page of the article must accompany payment. Consent does not extend to copying for general distribution, for promotion, for creating new works, or for resale. In these cases, specific written permission must be obtained from the copyright owner,
S. Karger AG,
P.O. Box, CH–4009 Basel (Switzerland).

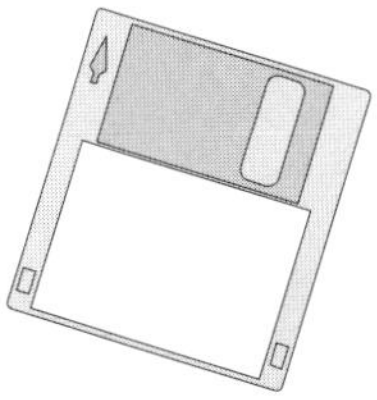

Disk Submission

A **comprehensive version** of these guidelines for the **submission of manuscripts and illustrations on disk** can be accessed online under **www.karger.com/journals/disksub.htm** or requested as a leaflet from the editorial department.

Please follow the general rules on style and arrangement in the **'Guidelines for Authors'** of the journal. Submit a **double-spaced printout** of your manuscript matching the file on disk exactly.

Technical Information
Store only data pertinent to this manuscript. Include your fonts (screen and printer fonts for Macintosh). For a **text only** manuscript, use a 3.5-inch disk. For **text and illustrations,** use 3.5 or 5.25 Magneto Optical Disc; CD-ROM (DOS or hybrid); iomage Zip/DOS (100 MB), or 44 MB, 88 MB or 200 MB SyQuest. Compress extensive data using ZIP format.

Data Description
Label your disk with the **title of the journal or book** for which it is submitted; a **short version** of the paper's title; your **name,** postal and e-mail address, fax and phone number; **hard and software** used, including the version; and the **complete list of the file names.** File names consist of eight characters before the dot identifying the file and three characters after the dot identifying the application.

Text and Format
The **preferred word-processing package is MS-Word.** Other commonly used PC text programs and ASCII formats are accepted.
Update your data when you revise subsequent to the reviewer's or editor's decision and mark revisions clearly. Manuscripts accepted for publication are subject to **copy editing:** changes and/or questions will be marked in the manuscript, which will be returned to you with your disk and the galley proofs for checking.
Enter your text continuously flush left. Do not use any layout functions. Do not split words at the end of a line. **Do not use indentations.** Use a blank line before and a hard return at the end of paragraphs.
Arrange headings flush left. Insert only **one space after punctuation marks.** Insert Greek letters, mathematical symbols etc. with your word-processing program. Use **boldface and italics** as well as sub- and superscript where appropriate.
Tables are part of the text and should be placed at the end of the text file. Separate the individual parts of a table by lines. Use the tabulator instead of spaces. Format operation data on one line in the same column. **Legends to illustrations are part of the text** and should also be listed at the end of the text file.

Illustrations
Store illustrations as separate files: do not integrate them in your text. Export **line drawings/vector graphics** as TIF, EPS or WMF format. Use Photoshop for processing and retouching **scanned halftone images.** Save the original scan and the processed version. Export **black and white or color images** as TIF or EPS format in their anticipated size in print. **For detailed information** on how to submit illustration data on disk please consult the leaflet or **www.karger.com/journals/disksub.htm.**

KARGER

KI 98 DISK

Fax+ 41 61 306 12 34
E-Mail karger@karger.ch
www.karger.com

The Journal Home Page is available at:
www.karger.com/journals/cto

Cells
Tissues
Organs

Moving Temporomandibular Joint Research into the 21st Century

Guest Editors
Arthur W. English, Atlanta, Ga.
Christian S. Stohler, Ann Arbor, Mich.

56 figures, 15 in color, 12 tables, 2001

KARGER

Basel · Freiburg · Paris · London · New York ·
New Delhi · Bangkok · Singapore · Tokyo · Sydney

S. Karger
Medical and Scientific Publishers
Basel · Freiburg · Paris · London
New York · New Delhi · Bangkok
Singapore · Tokyo · Sydney

Drug Dosage
The authors and the publisher have exerted every effort to ensure that drug selection and dosage set forth in this text are in accord with current recommendations and practice at the time of publication. However, in view of ongoing research, changes in government regulations, and the constant flow of information relating to drug therapy and drug reactions, the reader is urged to check the package insert for each drug for any change in indications and dosage and for added warnings and precautions. This is particularly important when the recommended agent is a new and/or infrequently employed drug.

P.O. Box, CH–4009 Basel (Switzerland)
Printed in Switzerland on acid-free paper by
Reinhardt Druck, Basel
ISBN 3–8055–7229–8

KARGER

Fax + 41 61 306 12 34
E-Mail karger@karger.ch
www.karger.com

Vol. 169, No. 3, 2001

Cells
Tissues
Organs

Contents

KARGER

Fax + 41 61 306 12 34
E-Mail karger@karger.ch
www.karger.com

Access to full text and tables of contents, including tentative ones for forthcoming issues:
www.karger.com/journals/cto/cto_bk.htm

Cells
Tissues
Organs

Cells Tissues Organs 2001;169:185–186

Preface

Patients suffering from temporomandibular joint (TMJ) disorders are a loosely defined group of individuals whose symptoms are characterized by pain, chiefly of musculoskeletal origin, in the head and neck region. In the general population, slightly more women are affected by these disorders than men, but among patients seeking medical attention at primary and even more at tertiary care centers, the overwhelming majority are females of childbearing age. Although the physical attributes appear to be similar between cases in primary and tertiary care settings, often remarkable differences with respect to severity, persistence, and impact exist between these patient populations. Significant case heterogeneity, including comorbid conditions, poses diagnostic difficulty in both research and clinical practice. There is currently no specific treatment for TMJ diseases and disorders. Patients suffering from these musculoskeletal pain conditions are often treated in questionable manners using strategies that have little or no science base.

The Milwaukee-based patient advocacy group, The TMJ Association, a non-profit-making foundation founded in 1986 (www.tmj.org), with co-sponsorship by the National Institutes of Allergy and Infectious Diseases, Child Health and Human Development, Dental and Craniofacial Research, and Neurological Disorders and Stroke, and the Office of Research on Women's Health brought together over 30 scientists to explore and discuss topics relevant to the understanding of craniofacial pain and jaw dysfunction, as manifested in temporomandibular joint diseases and disorders. The Workshop, entitled: 'Moving TMJ Research into the 21st Century' was held at the Conference Center of the Federation of American Societies of Experimental Biology in Bethesda, Md., May 22–23, 2000. Experts in arthritis, TMJ pathology, bone, joint, and muscle physiology, neurobiology, pain, genetics, endocrinology, immunology, wound healing and tissue engineering presented papers and engaged in working groups, charged to identify the immediate and long-range research needs that will advance the understanding of the etiopathogenesis of TMJ injury and diseases that will ultimately lead to evidence-based treatments for these conditions. Nearly half of the participants work in the head and neck field on subjects directly related to TMJ diseases and disorders, while the other scientists focus on research questions outside of the craniofacial complex. Because of the quality of the papers and the high level of scientific interchange they fostered, all who participated in the first annual meeting of the TMJ Association considered it a success. The goal of the organizers, to get people together and get them exchanging ideas, was met.

After the first day of oral presentations, workshop participants engaged in productive discussions, defining critical future research directions, including the specific obstacles that hinder progress in this field. Participants called for animal, cell culture and computer models to study the intact, injured and diseased TMJ; the development of diagnostic taxonomies based on mechanistic understanding of TMJ pain, inflammation and degeneration; the characterization of the clinical disease spectrum using advanced biotechnologies; the study of the biomechanics of the intact, injured and diseased TMJ; research on the maturation, adaptation, and response to TMJ inju-

KARGER
Fax + 41 61 306 12 34
E-Mail karger@karger.ch
www.karger.com

1422–6405/01/1693–0185$17.50/0

Accessible online at:
www.karger.com/journals/cto

ry and disease, including the unique tissue repair problems in TMJ patients. Additional areas of needed research include the screening of existing transgenic models for the presence of TMJ pathology, the exploration of novel reconstruction methodologies, including the potential of protein and gene therapy for TMJ pain and repair.

Papers presented during the first day of the meeting are included in this special issue of *Cells, Tissues, Organs.* The diversity of their topics and their synthetic approach form the type of papers that we hope will become the standard in *Cells, Tissues, Organs.* We thank the authors for their dedication and hard work and hope that this volume will reflect a comprehensive state-of-the-art summary of basic research related to TMJ diseases and disorders. We are delighted to be able to present this special topics issue, 'New Perspectives on Temporomandibular Disorders', as a complete number of *Cells, Tissues, Organs.* It represents the breadth of science that appears in the journal and, especially, our areas of focus on tissue engineering artificial organs, in vitro systems, and integrative neuroscience. We hope that this issue of the journal will be useful to scientists both in and out of the TMJ field, and to patients and their advocates as well.

Arthur W. English, Atlanta, Ga.
Christian S. Stohler, Ann Arbor, Mich.

Cells
Tissues
Organs

Cells Tissues Organs 2001;169:187–192

Temporomandibular Disorders and Hormones in Women

Michelle P. Warren Joanna L. Fried

Departments of Medicine and Obstetrics and Gynecology, Columbia College of Physicians and Surgeons, New York, N.Y., USA

Key Words

Temporomandibular joint · Temporomandibular disorder · Hormones · Women

Abstract

Temporomandibular disorders (TMD) are loosely defined as an assorted set of clinical conditions, characterized by pain and dysfunction of the masticatory system. Pain in the masticatory muscles, in the temporomandibular joint (TMJ), and in associated hard and soft tissues, limitation in jaw function, and sounds in the TMJ are common symptoms. That women make up the majority of patients treated for TMD is extensively hypothesized and documented in numerous epidemiological studies. Certain contradictory studies exist which propose that there are no statistically significant gender differences in the actual incidence of changes in joint morphology. Nonetheless, extensive literature suggests the disorder is 1.5–2 times more prevalent in women than in men, and that 80% of patients treated for TMD are women. The severity of symptoms is also related to the age of the patients. Pain onset tends to occur after puberty, and peaks in the reproductive years, with the highest prevalence occurring in women aged 20–40, and the lowest among children, adolescents, and the elderly. The gender and age distribution of TMD suggests a possible link between its pathogenesis and the female hormonal axis. In this review, we will use the hypothesis that the overwhelming majority of patients treated for temporomandibular disorders are women and use the available literature to examine the role of hormones in TMD.

Temporomandibular disorders (TMD) are loosely defined as an assorted set of clinical conditions, characterized by pain and dysfunction of the masticatory system. Pain in the masticatory muscles, in the temporomandibular joint (TMJ), and in associated hard and soft tissues, limitation in jaw function, and sound in the TMJ are common symptoms [Kuttila et al., 1998].

That women make up the majority of patients treated for TMD is extensively hypothesized and documented in numerous epidemiological studies [Campbell et al., 1993; Koidis et al., 1993; Jagger et al., 1994; Carlsson and LeResche, 1995; Abubaker et al., 1996; LeResche et al., 1997]. Certain contradictory studies exist which propose that there are no statistically significant gender differences in the actual incidence of changes in joint morphology [Helkimo, 1976; Widmalm et al., 1994]. Nonetheless, extensive literature suggests the disorder is 1.5–2 times

KARGER

Fax + 41 61 306 12 34
E-Mail karger@karger.ch
www.karger.com

1422–6405/01/1693–0187$17.50/0

Accessible online at:
www.karger.com/journals/cto

Michelle P. Warren, MD
Department of Ob/Gyn, PH 16–20, Columbia University
622 West 168th Street
New York, NY 10032 (USA)
Tel. +1 212 305 8723, Fax +1 212 305 9945, E-Mail mpwl@columbia.edu

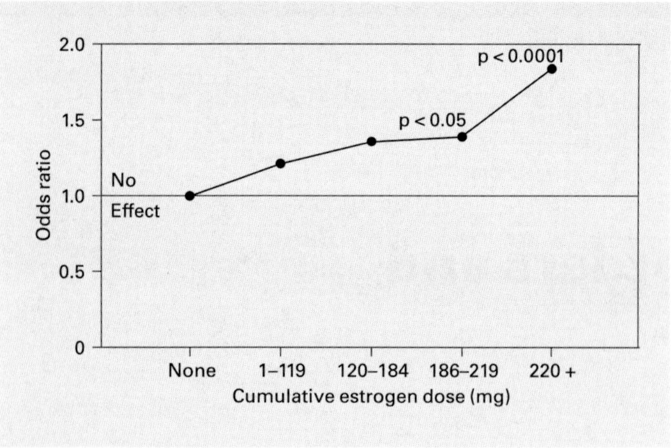

Fig. 1. Risk of TMD (odds ratio) by level of cumulative estrogen exposure in the year prior to index date (controlled for health services use). Reproduced with permission from the International Association for the Study of Pain [LeResche et al., 1997].

more prevalent in women than in men, and that 80% of patients treated for TMD are women [LeResche, 1997; Kapila and Xie, 1998]. The severity of symptoms is also related to the age of the patients. Pain onset tends to occur after puberty, and peaks in the reproductive years [Meisler, 1999], with the highest prevalence occurring in women aged 20–40 years, and the lowest among children, adolescents, and the elderly [Kuttila et al., 1998].

In examining any disease or disorder that displays a sex predilection, it is important to address three possible causal factors. The first is the biological and physiological differences that might cause one sex to be more vulnerable to the disease or disorder. The second is the behavioral factors which might lead to the gender distinction. And the third consideration is genetic; to what extent do genetic factors associated with sex account for the discrepancy in incidence? In examining the hypothesis that the overwhelming majority of patients treated for temporomandibular disorders (TMD) are women, we will look at each of these three factors.

The gender and age distribution of TMD suggests a possible link between its pathogenesis and the female reproductive system. As early as 1986, numerous estrogen receptors were found in the temporomandibular joint complex of female baboons [Aufdemorte et al., 1986]. More recently, several studies have shown the presence of high-affinity estrogen receptors in the articular cartilage of humans. Further, in a very limited study of the TMJ specimens of 14 women and 8 men, estrogen and progesterone receptors were found in varying frequencies in both symptomatic and asymptomatic women and men [Abubaker et al., 1993]. However, the authors of a similar 1993 study came to the conclusion that TMD may not be hormonally modulated by estrogens, when the study of 14 human TMJ samples revealed no significant presence of estrogen receptors in the tissue [Campbell et al., 1993]. More recently, a study of castrated rats indicated that steroid sex hormones do have an effect on the collagen and protein content of the TMJ disc; its authors conclude that the collagen content of the TMJ disc in the normal rat is dependent on the animal's sex [Abubaker et al., 1996].

Collagen and elastin make up a great deal of the temporomandibular joint disc's structure, and are often found to be altered in the presence of TMD symptoms. The direct influence of sex hormones on changes in collagen and elastin synthesis is well established, and there is a great deal of evidence that sex steroids have a direct metabolic effect on cartilage cells [Corvol et al., 1992]. Clinical studies have shown that there are estrogen receptors in human knee joints, and that the level of estradiol in the synovial fluid correlates to the severity of osteoarthritis in these joints [Dworkin et al., 1990]. In 1996, one study found that steroid sex hormones have an effect on the collagen and protein content of the TMJ disc [Abubaker et al., 1996]. In addition to the effect on cartilage, estrogen and progesterone may have significant effects on bone.

Several studies have examined exogenous hormone use and the risk of TMD among postmenopausal women. A 1997 audit of the records of a large health maintenance organization found that the use of exogenous estrogen significantly increased the odds of having TMD, a risk that increases with higher doses of estrogen (fig. 1). This study also reported that the odds of being a TMD case were approximately 30% higher among women receiving estrogen compared to those not exposed, and concluded that the use of oral contraceptives was associated with an increased risk of approximately 20% [LeResche et al., 1997] (tables 1, 2). Another study reported a higher prevalence of use of birth control pills, estrogen, and progesterone among women with TMD symptoms compared to women of the same age without symptoms [Abubaker et al., 1992].

It is important to note, however, that the studies involving exogenous hormones were conducted during a time when hormone replacement therapy, in particular estrogen replacement therapy, was offered primarily to women who had undergone a hysterectomy. A 1995 survey of 495 postmenopausal women concluded that having undergone hysterectomy was the characteristic most strongly associated with hormone replacement therapy

Table 1. Prediction of case/control status: estrogen replacement therapy and health service use (n = 987 TMD cases, 3,948 controls)

Variable	Odds ratio (95% CI)	χ^2	p
Controlled by age			
Use of estrogen replacements	1.64 (1.38–1.94)	33.0	<0.001
Controlled by age and health services use			
Use of estrogen replacements	1.32 (1.10–1.57)	9.3	0.002
Number of medical and surgical visits in prior year	2.75 (2.60–2.91)	318.9	<0.001

Reproduced with permission from the International Association for the Study of Pain [LeResche et al., 1997].

Table 2. Prediction of case/control status: oral contraceptive and health service use (n = 979 TMD cases, 3,916 controls)

Variable	Odds ratio (95% CI)	χ^2	p
Controlled by age			
Oral contraceptive use	1.632 (1.12–1.54)	11.6	<0.001
Controlled by age and health services use			
Oral contraceptive use	1.19 (1.01–1.40)	4.3	0.04
Number of medical and surgical visits in prior year	1.94 (1.84–2.04)	168.2	<0.001

Reproduced with permission from the International Association for the Study of Pain [LeResche et al., 1997].

use. This study found that 37.6% of the women surveyed reported use of hormone replacement therapy and that it was used by 58.7% of women who had undergone a hysterectomy and 19.6% of women who had not (p = 0.001) [Keating et al., 1999]. There has been no investigation of the correlation between hysterectomies and TMD. Hysterectomized women have been found to have higher rates of osteoarthritis than controls, suggesting a possible link between hysterectomy and joint and/or chronic pain disorders [Spector et al., 1991]. Additionally, the surgery itself could have any number of effects on the temporomandibular joint and pain transmission. The effects of general anesthesia and endotracheal intubation on the pathogenesis of pain and the morphology of the temporomandibular joint have not been investigated.

Some studies examining the effects of hormones on TMD have been contradictory. One study found that women with TMD reported higher use of exogenous hormones than controls [Abubaker et al., 1993], while another proposed that there may be an inverse relationship between circulating estrogen levels and joint pain [Haskin et al., 1995]. The role of female sex hormones in the pathogenesis of TMD has been a source of controversy. It has been proposed that the contradictory results of research on sex hormones and TMD may indicate that while excessive exogenous ovarian hormones can put a woman at risk for TMD, the endogenous hormones are essential for the remodeling of the TMJ [Yasuoka et al., 2000].

Another possible hormonal factor may be relaxin, a female polypeptide hormone produced by the corpus luteum. It is present in the blood in the last days of the menstrual cycle prior to the onset of menstruation and throughout pregnancy [Chamberlain and Broughton-Pipkin, 1998], and it is thought to cause muscle relaxation during childbirth. It is also a known modulator of tissue-remodeling activity in the female reproductive organs. Increased systemic joint laxity in pregnant women has been linked to elevated levels of relaxin. Relaxin levels increase 2- to 3-fold during pregnancy. A 1998 study found that relaxin increases the expression of specific tissue-degrading enzymes. While the authors of this study acknowledge that hormones like relaxin do not fully explain the gender and age distribution of TMD, they propose that it may predispose women to aberrant joint remodeling by modulating the expression of matrix-degrading enzymes [Kapila and Xie, 1998]. However, a 1988 study found that women with TMD have a significantly lower natality than women without the disorder, and have higher rates of premenstrually related pain symptoms [Marbach et al., 1988].

Another effect of estrogen may be to increase the synthesis of cytokines, proteins secreted by inflammatory leukocytes and some non-leukocytic cells which act as intercellular mediators and which have been implicated in degenerative diseases. Cytokines may be involved in remodeling and degenerative activities affecting the TMJ [Haskin et al., 1995].

Finally, there is the uncertain role of female sex hormones in pain transmission. Even if there are no significant physiological differences in the TMJs of men and women, it is possible that women experience the disorder more acutely than men, thus being more likely to seek treatment. In addition to increasing the presence of cytokines, estrogen may down-regulate the synthesis of prostaglandins, which would lead to an inverse relationship between circulating estrogen levels and pain in the joint [Haskin et al., 1995].

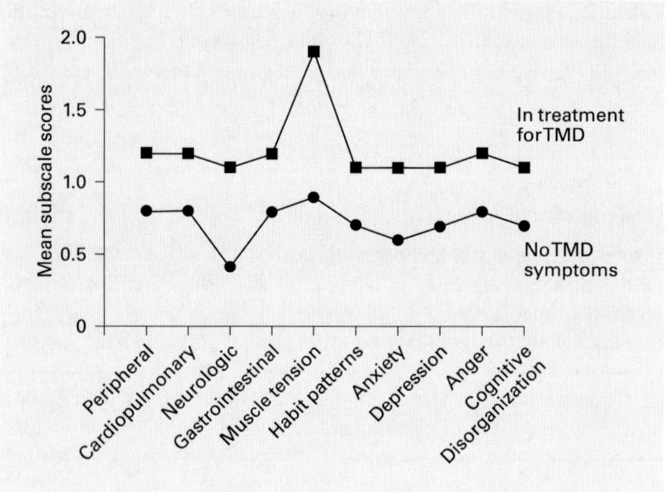

Fig. 2. Mean scores from the Symptoms of Stress Inventory subscales. Reproduced with permission from Quintessence Publishing Co., Inc. [Kuttila et al., 1998].

A final consideration of the potentially gender-specific physiological pathogenesis is ergonomic. It has been suggested that men generally tend to experience more musculoskeletal pain in the lower back while women are more likely to present with complaints in the neck, arms, and shoulders [Krogstad et al., 1996a].

A significant amount of research effort has been spent on drawing links between psychological factors and the occurrence/severity of TMD. Much research has focused on the correlations between TMD and high levels of stress and/or depression [Carlsson et al., 1982; Kuttila et al., 1998]. A 1998 study reported that women showed higher total stress scores on a standardized Symptoms of Stress Inventory than men. Female TMD patients showed significantly higher stress scores in terms of muscle tension [Kuttila et al., 1998] (fig. 2). It is also suggested that anxiety may be an important factor in the perception of pain, and that a reduction in anxiety levels may lead to more effective treatment response and/or more pain tolerance for TMD patients [Krogstad et al., 1996b]. Some recent data indicate that there is little to no support for the hypothesis that stress and psychological state have a significant effect on treatment outcome [Wexler and Steed, 1998]. Psychological factors may indeed play a part in TMD, and the incidence of depression and related disorders is traditionally higher in women. However, a more thorough examination of the physiological aspects of the disease, especially as it relates to gender, must be pursued before any conclusions can be drawn.

Another behavioral factor which might influence the incidence of TMD in women is women's use of health services. Research has shown that gender is an important predictor of medical care utilization. It has been argued that women use more medical services because they are more sensitive to symptoms and more interested in health than men; another theory is that women's greater service utilization arises from the fact that women experience more morbidities than do men [Green and Pope, 1999]. Women may be more familiar and comfortable with pain reporting and may be more comfortable in the role of patient [Krogstad et al., 1996a], and may also be more persistent in seeking treatment in the face of treatment failures [Marbach et al., 1997]. Regardless of the possible psychological processes involved, studies of health behavior in adults do show that women report more morbidity in addition to greater health service utilization than do men, despite lower mortality rates [Rudolf et al., 1992].

A further gender difference is found in the treatment of TMD. A study of one insurance company's records of people with TMD-related diagnoses (n = 46,293) found that females were 2–3 times more likely than males to undergo surgical as opposed to nonsurgical treatment for TMD. This suggests that women are more likely to seek or be recommended for this surgical procedure, which is as yet of undetermined safety and efficacy [Marbach et al., 1997].

Another possible behavioral factor which might be explored is women's relationship to eating and to food. A 1999 study reported that women were more likely than men to report weight control behaviors, with particularly strong associations found between gender and 'history of dieting' (odds ratio = 8.1) and 'participation in an organized weight loss program' (odds ratio = 11.7) [Neumark-Sztainer et al., 1999]. These factors have not been examined in relationship to TMD in women.

An avenue which merits further exploration combines biological and behavioral factors; a 1999 study identified *Chlamydia trachomatis* in the TMJ. Thirty-nine percent (all women) of 30 TMD patients (29 women, 2 men) had *C. trachomatis* present in TMJ tissue. There is a well-established connection between STDs and reactive arthritis. Sexually active women under the age of 20 are at the highest risk for chlamydial infection [Henry et al., 1999]. Chlamydia infections may be dormant and asymptomatic for months or even years, and many women are infected and do not know it. While the above study had a very small sample and no control group, it presents yet another underexamined area of TMD research.

The third consideration, that of the possible role of sex chromosomes in the incidence of TMD, has not been specifically explored. The genetic basis for sex-linked diseases has long been the subject of investigation; in 1995, Holmdahl found that the female preponderance for development of arthritis in rats is influenced by both sex chromosomes and sex steroids [Holmdahl, 1995]. While significant research energy has gone into (and should continue to go into) the roles of women's hormones and habits in the incidence of TMD, the role of genetics is another important area that must be addressed.

Despite the intriguing results of a handful of studies, there is not sufficient research to support any conclusions about the gender difference in the occurrence of TMD. While some research has pointed out that degenerative joint disease occurs more frequently in women than in men, others have reported that despite differences in pain, there are no statistically significant gender differences in the actual incidence of changes in joint morphology. Furthermore, no studies have addressed other possible sources of joint damage. Many women on exogenous hormones have undergone hysterectomies. Is there any correlation between surgery and the incidence of TMD? Are there direct connections between the age of onset of menstruation or menopause and that of TMD? Is it possible that equal numbers of women and men actually have joint displacement or degeneration, but that women experience more pain, report it more often, or are referred for it more frequently? Chronic pain problems are complex to treat due to their multidimensional natures. There are numerous factors beyond the physiological which play important roles, such as disparities in health-care access and/or usage, somatization, and the diversity of responses to treatment.

It seems that two issues are at play in terms of the proposed high incidence of TMD in women. The first is whether women are more at risk for the one of the varied physiological factors thought to cause TMD (internal derangement of the temporomandibular joint, displacement of the disc between the condyle and the temporal bone, arthritis of the jaw joint, etc.). The second is whether women, due to either psychological, hormonal, or chromosomal factors, experience more significant pain or discomfort due to the disorder. As LeResche et al. [1997] propose, reproductive hormones may act centrally to influence pain neurotransmission.

As of today, there is not enough research into any one of these possible avenues. There exist too many factors to draw meaningful conclusions as to why (or even, possibly, *if*) more TMD cases are women. Furthermore, TMD itself is not a clearly enough defined diagnosis, but more a catchall phrase for pain, discomfort, and/or disability associated with the temporomandibular joint. With the three factors of biology, behavior, and genetics in mind, this is a women's health issue demanding further exploration and explanation.

References

Abubaker, A.O., P.C. Hebda, J.N. Gunsolley (1996) Effects of sex hormones on protein and collagen content of the temporomandibular joint disc of the rat. J Oral Maxillofac Surg *54:* 721–727.

Abubaker, A.O., F. John, G.C. Sotereanos, G. Patterson, J. Jenosky (1992) Prevalence of female sex hormone use by female TMJ patients. J Dent Res *71:* 259 (abstract).

Abubaker, A.O., W.F. Raslan, G.C. Sotereanos (1993) Estrogen and progesterone receptors in temporomandibular joint discs of symptomatic and asymptomatic persons: A preliminary study. J Oral Maxillofac Surg *51:* 1096–1100.

Aufdemorte, T.B., J.E. Van Sickels, M.F. Dolwick, P.J. Sheridan, G.R. Holt, S.B. Aragon (1986) Estrogen receptors in the temporomandibular joint of the baboon *(Papio cynocephalus:* An autoradiographic study. Oral Surg Oral Med Oral Pathol *61:* 307–314.

Campbell, J.H., M.S. Courey, P. Bourne, C. Odziemiec (1993) Estrogen receptor analysis of human temporomandibular disc. J Oral Maxillofac Surg *51:* 1101–1105.

Carlsson, G.E., S. Kopp, A. Wedel (1982) Analysis of background variables in 350 patients with TMJ disorders as reported in self administered questionnaire. Commun Dent Oral Epidemiol *10:* 47–51.

Carlsson, G.E., L. LeResche (1995) Epidemiology of temporomandibular disorders; in Sessle, B.J., P.S. Bryant, R.A. Dionne (eds): Temporomandibular Disorder and Related Pain Conditions. Seattle, IASP Press, vol 4, pp 211–226.

Chamberlain, G., F. Broughton-Pipkin (1998) Clinical Physiology in Obstetrics. Malden, Blackwell Science.

Corvol, M., O. Blanchard, L. Tsagris (1992) Bone and cartilage responsiveness to sex steroid hormones. J Steroid Biochem Mol Biol *43:* 415–418.

Dworkin, S.F., K.H. Huggins, L. LeResche, M. Von Korff, J. Howard, E. Truelove, E. Sommers (1990) Epidemiology of signs and symptoms in temporomandibular disorders: Clinical signs in cases and controls. J Am Dent Assoc *120:* 273–281.

Green, C.A., C.R. Pope (1999) Gender, psychosocial factors and the use of medical services: A longitudinal analysis. Soc Sci Med *48:* 1363–1372.

Haskin, C.L., S.B. Milam, I.L. Cameron (1995) Pathogenesis of degenerative joint disease in the human temporomandibular joint. Crit Rev Oral Biol Med *6:* 248–277.

Helkimo, M. (1976) Epidemiological surveys of dysfunction of the masticatory system. Oral Sci Rev *7:* 54–69.

Henry, C.H., A.P. Hudson, H.C. Gerard, P.F. Franco, L.M. Wolford (1999) Identification of *Chlamydia trachomatis* in the human temporomandibular joint. J Oral Maxillofac Surg *57:* 683–688.

Holmdahl, R. (1995) Female preponderance for development of arthritis in rats is influenced by both sex chromosomes and sex steroids. Scand J Immunol *42:* 104–109.

Jagger, R.G., J.F. Bates, S. Kopp (1994) Temporomandibular Joint Dysfunction. Oxford, Wright.

Kapila, S., Y. Xie (1998) Targeted induction of collagenase and stromelysin by relaxin in unprimed and beta-estradiol-primed diarthrodial joint fibrocartilaginous cells but not in synoviocytes. Lab Invest *78:* 925–938.

Keating, N.L., P.D. Cleary, A.S. Rossi, A.M. Zaslavsky, J.Z. Ayanian (1999) Use of hormone replacement therapy by postmenopausal women in the United States (see comments). Ann Intern Med *130:* 545–553.

Koidis, P.T., A. Zarifi, E. Grigoriadou, P. Garefis (1993) Effect of age and sex on craniomandibular disorders. J Prosthet Dent *69:* 93–101.

Krogstad, B.S., A. Jokstad, B.L. Dahl, O. Vassend (1996a) The reporting of pain, somatic complaints, and anxiety in a group of patients with TMD before and 2 years after treatment: Sex differences. J Orofac Pain *10:* 263–269.

Krogstad, B.S., A. Jokstad, B.L. Dahl, O. Vassend (1996b) Relationships between risk factors and treatment outcome in a group of patients with temporomandibular disorders. J Orofac Pain *10:* 48–53.

Kuttila, M., P.M. Niemi, S. Kuttila, P. Alanen, Y. Le Bell (1998) TMD treatment need in relation to age, gender, stress, and diagnostic subgroup. J Orofac Pain *12:* 67–74.

LeResche, L (1997) Epidemiology of temporomandibular disorders: Implications for the investigation of etiologic factors. Crit Rev Oral Biol Med *8:* 291–305.

LeResche, L., K. Saunders, M.R. Von Korff, W. Barrlow, S.F. Dworking (1997) Use of exogenous hormones and risk of temporomandibular disorder pain. Pain *69:* 153–160.

Marbach, J.J., G.T. Ballard, M.R. Frankel, K.G. Raphael (1997) Patterns of TMJ surgery: Evidence of sex differences (see comments). J Am Dent Assoc *128:* 609–614.

Marbach, J.J., M.C. Lennon, B.P. Dohrenwend (1988) Candidate risk factors for temporomandibular pain and dysfunction syndrome: Psychosocial, health behavior, physical illness and injury. Pain *34:* 139–151.

Meisler, J.G. (1999) Chronic pain conditions in women. J Womens Health *8:* 313–320.

Neumark-Sztainer, D., N.E. Sherwood, S.A. French, R.W. Jeffery (1999) Weight control behaviors among adult men and women: Cause for concern? Obes Res *7:* 179–188.

Rudolf, M.C., O. Tomanovich, J. Greenberg, L. Friend, A.J. Alario (1992) Gender differences in infirmary use at a residential summer camp. J Dev Behav Pediatr *13:* 261–265.

Spector, T.D., D.J. Hart, P. Brown, J. Almeyda, J.E. Dacre, D.V. Doyle, A.J. Silman (1991) Frequency of osteoarthritis in hysterectomized women. J Rheumatol *18:* 1877–1883.

Wexler, G.B., P.A. Steed (1998) Psychological factors and temporomandibular outcomes. Cranio *16:* 72–77.

Widmalm, S.E., P.L. Westesson, I.K. Kim, F.J. Pereira Jr., H. Lundh, M.M. Tasaki (1994) Temporomandibular joint pathosis related to sex, age, and dentition in autopsy material. Oral Surg Oral Med Oral Pathol *78:* 416–425.

Yasuoka, T., M. Nakashima, T. Okuda, N. Tatematsu (2000) Effect of estrogen replacement on temporomandibular joint remodeling in ovariectomized rats. J Oral Maxillofac Surg *58:* 189–196.

masseter muscle insertion forward, but because the origin of the masseter stays at the skull, the muscle's action line falls further behind the bite point than before. This change in geometry should increase, not decrease, the reaction loading on the condyle. Clearly, the situation is more complex than a simple lever analysis! The complicating factors probably include (1) muscle length-tension relationships, and (2) joint contact areas. With regard to the muscle, the masseter is shortened by protrusion, and therefore probably produced less force [Anapol and Herring, 1989]. With regard to the joint, extensive protrusion may lessen the contact between the condyle and the articular eminence, causing the load to be dissipated by soft tissue distortion. Although the apparent unloading of the protruded TMJ seems to support the use of anterior repositioning splints in patients, longer term (two months) use of such devices actually led to condylar pathology [Sindelar et al., 2000], perhaps because of the limitations that splints place on jaw movement.

Peak Loads Are Not the Only Loads

Mastication is not a static activity. Strains are caused by muscles, but chewing is a complex choreography of muscle contraction. Bone strains are therefore dynamic. For example, strains in the skull vault can veer between tension and compression several times in a single masticatory cycle [Herring and Teng, 2000]. The TMJ is no exception. Although peak masticatory strains are strongly compressive, smaller, tensile strains occasionally occur. In figure 4, peak strains (arrowheads in 4A and dashed lines in 4B) show compression oriented postero-superiorly to antero-inferiorly, but a secondary pattern can be seen just before the second chewing cycle. In this secondary pattern (small arrows in 4A and solid lines in 4B), it is tension that is observed in the postero-superior to antero-inferior direction. Interestingly, this secondary strain corresponds to early activity in the left (contralateral) masseter muscle (fig. 4A). A similar pattern of tension occurs in anesthetized pigs when the contralateral masseter is stimulated (fig. 2B). A likely explanation for this phenomenon is an asymmetrical mandibular rotation set up by unilateral masseter contraction (fig. 4C) as proposed by other authors [Crompton and Hylander, 1986; Dessem and Druzinsky, 1992]. The practical importance of this finding is that TMJ prostheses must have some tensile strength even though the major load is compressive.

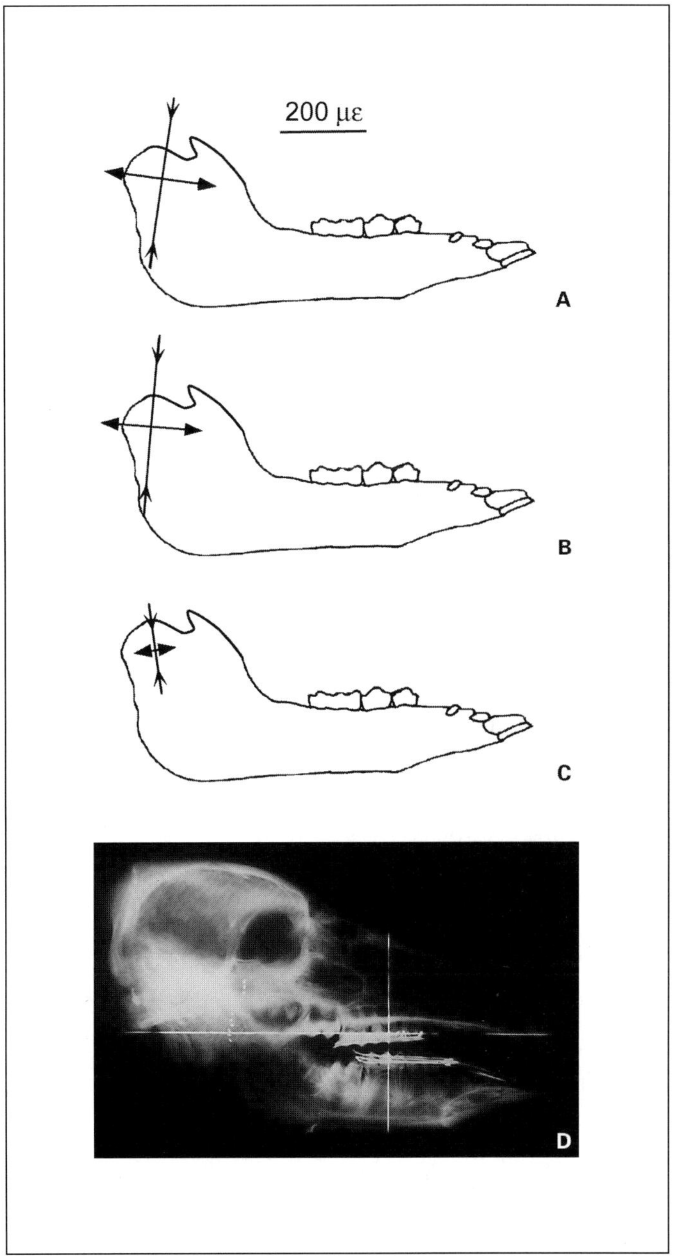

Fig. 3. An example of the alteration of condylar strain by repositioning the mandible. Adapted from Marks et al. [1997]. Bilateral stimulation of masseter and temporalis muscles with occlusal splints holding the mandible in various positions. Arrows pointing toward the gage site indicate compressive strain, while those pointing away indicate tension. **A** Resting position with teeth separated from centric occlusion by the splint. **B** Retruded 2.5 mm from (**A**). **C** Protruded 6.75 mm from (**A**). **D** Radiograph of a head with the splints luted in the protrusive position. Resting and retruded positions produced identical strains to centric occlusion, but strains were reduced in protrusion.

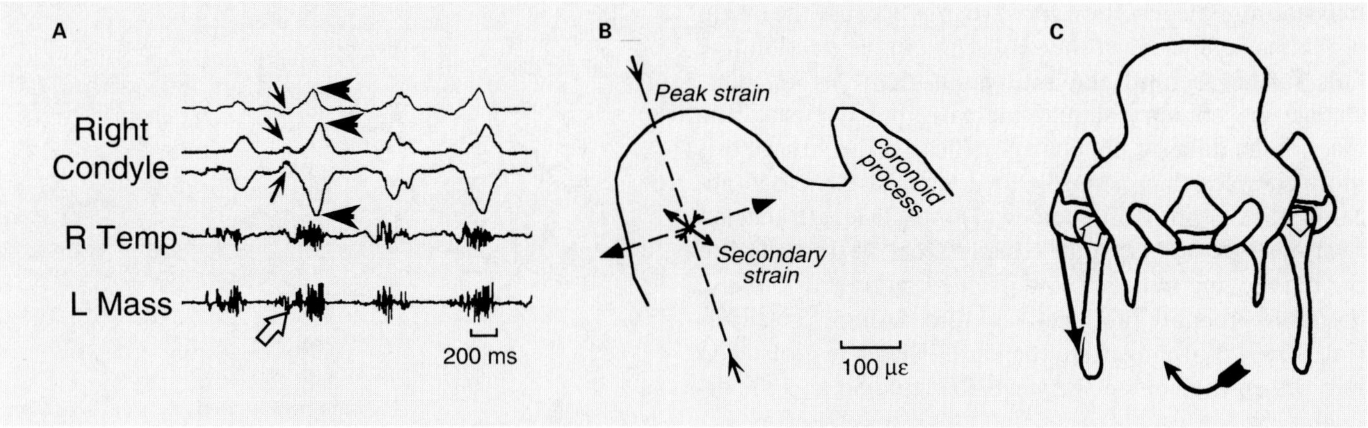

Fig. 4. Dynamic changes in condylar strain during mastication in a young pig. Adapted from Herring and Mucci [1991] and Herring [1998]. **A** Raw strain from the three elements of the stacked rosette strain gage on the right condylar neck and EMG from the right temporalis (R Temp) and left masseter (L Mass) muscles. Four masticatory cycles are seen. The moment of peak strain for the second cycle is indicated by the arrowheads. A preceding, much smaller strain peak is indicated by small arrows; it corresponds with an early burst from the contralateral (left) masseter (open arrow). **B** Principal strains calculated from the raw strains in (**A**), conventions as in figure 3. Although the peak strains (dashed arrows) are compressive, in the secondary pattern (solid arrows), tension is larger. **C** Suggested mechanism for the secondary strain pattern. Unilateral contraction of the left masseter (black arrow) sets up an asymmetric rotation of mandible, such that the left TMJ is compressed but the right (instrumented) condyle comes away from the skull (open arrows).

The Cranial Element of the TMJ Shows Tension, Not Compression

The most surprising result of the strain gage studies was that the location just lateral to the articular eminence is under an entirely different strain regime than the lateral surface of the condyle. Specifically, tension, oriented from postero-superior to antero-inferior, greatly exceeds compression (fig. 5), [Liu and Herring, 2000b]. Although this strain is strikingly different from condylar strain, it is of similar magnitude (averaging +212 με and –72 με for principal strains) and comes from the same source, contraction of the ipsilateral masseter [Liu and Herring, 2000a].

The surprising difference in strain pattern between the condyle and the squamosal bone does not mean that different forces are imposed on the two bony elements of the joint. On the contrary, the forces on the articulating surfaces must be the same and almost certainly are compressive. However, whereas the relatively simple condyle receives the load almost along the long axis of the mandibular ramus, the irregularly shaped squamosal bone is loaded at various projections, causing bending and torsion. Specifically, the pull of the masseter bends the entire zygomatic process of the squamosal such that the lateral side becomes more convex and the medial side more concave [Rafferty et al., 2000]. At the same time, in pigs the articular eminence is not buttressed by the braincase as in humans, but juts laterally, where compression from the condyle probably bends it like a cantilever beam (fig. 6), [Teng et al., 1997].

Thus, the same TMJ forces that load the condyle in almost axial compression instead bend and twist the articular eminence. This difference underscores a fundamental point about the biomechanics of the skull, the fact that stress and strain in the tissues depend as much on geometry as they do on the applied forces.

The Architecture of the TMJ Bones Reflects Their Strain Regimes

Axial compression and bending cause very different patterns of stress transmission. Axial loads are borne by the entire cross-section of a structure, whereas bending leads to high stresses peripherally but little or no stress in the interior [Wainwright, 1988]. For this reason, bones that are loaded axially or in shear (e.g. vertebral bodies) have very little cortex, but instead are composed of evenly distributed trabecular bone. The trabeculae are typically in rough alignment with the compressive and/or tensile stress [Martin et al., 1998]. In contrast, bones that are loaded in bending or in torsion (e.g. long bones including the body of the mandible) feature a thick cortex of compact bone and a central area with few trabeculae or just a marrow cavity.

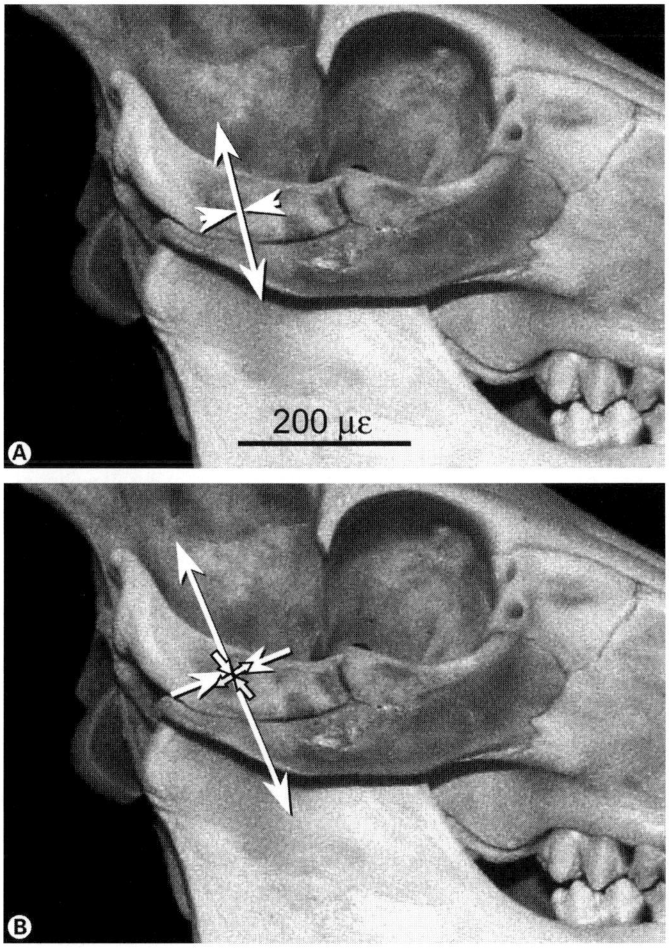

Fig. 5. Average principal strains on the squamosal bone. **A** Peak strains during mastication. Adapted from Liu and Herring [2000b]. Tension predominates. **B** Strains during stimulation of the ipsilateral (large arrows) and contralateral (small arrows) masseter. Adapted from Liu and Herring [2000a]. As for the condyle, the ipsilateral masseter produces the same pattern as mastication, but the contralateral masseter does not.

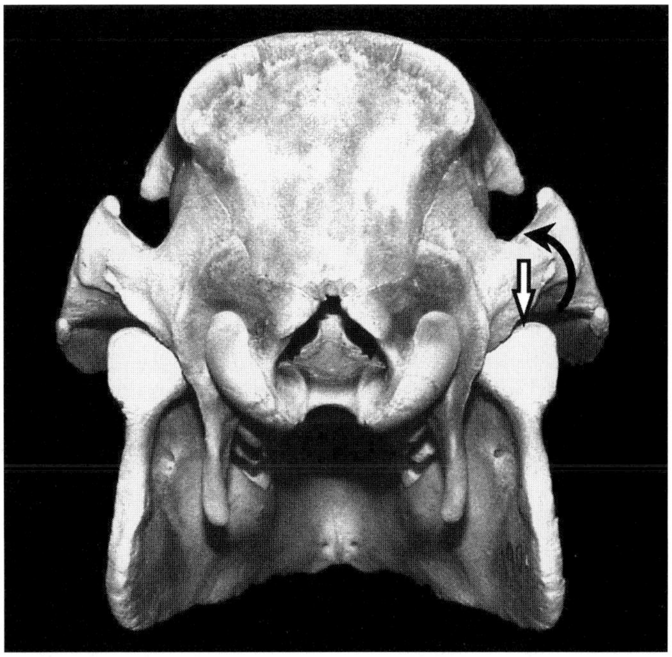

Fig. 6. Diagram indicating how the condyle can be compressed while the articular eminence is bent as a cantilever.

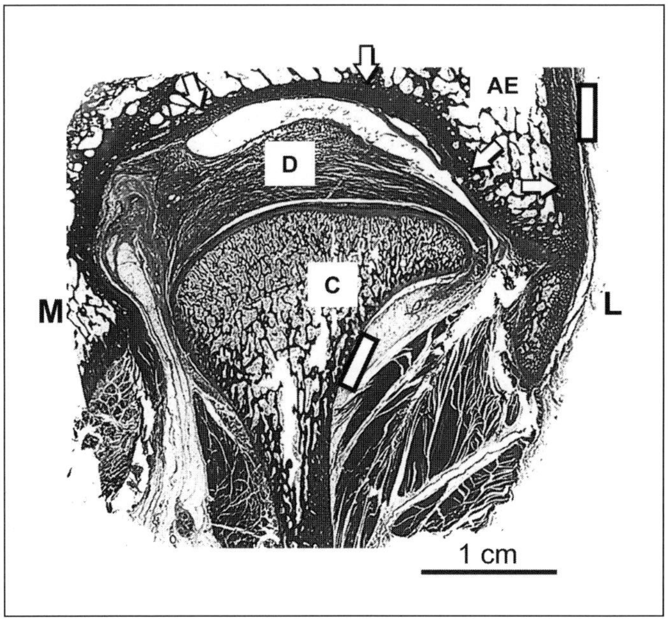

Fig. 7. Histological section in the frontal plane through the TMJ of a 10-month-old miniature pig. HE. AE = Articular eminence; C = mandibular condyle; D = TMJ disc, sectioned through the posterior band; L = lateral; M = medial. The white rectangles show the approximate position of the strain gages. The arrows indicate the compact cortical bone of the articular eminence; the condyle has little or no cortex, but is filled with fine trabeculae.

Figure 7 shows a frontal section through a pig TMJ. It is quite clear that the internal structure of the condyle and articular eminence differ. The head of the condyle is composed almost entirely of fine cancellous bone; there is little cortical bone until relatively far down onto the condylar neck. Furthermore, the alignment of the trabeculae is strongly superior-inferior. Quantitative analysis of sections taken in different planes confirms this vertical orientation and indicates a secondary orientation in the parasagittal plane [Teng and Herring, 1995]. The condyle is therefore composed of perforated bony plates arranged antero-posteriorly. Such a structure can line up with a compressive load applied at any parasagittal angle, and indeed the condyle is stronger and stiffer under compression applied in the superior-inferior direction than in any other plane [Teng and Herring, 1996]. In contrast, the articular eminence has relatively few trabeculae, and the bulk of its bony tissue is compact cortical bone (fig. 7). This distribution of bone implies bending or torsion, as does the fact that the few trabeculae present tend to be arranged from medial to lateral rather than from superior to inferior [Teng et al., 1997].

The demonstration in pigs of a correlation between loading and internal architecture will help in the extrapolation of these results to the human condition, which cannot be assessed directly. Pigs are too different from humans to allow us to assume that all the present results can be applied directly to the clinical situation. However, it is reasonable to assume that bony architecture reflects loading in any mammal, including humans. With modern techniques such as X-ray tomography, it will be possible to assess variations in trabecular architecture in living individuals and even to track longitudinal changes in single individuals [Odgaard, 1997]. In this way, we can hope to learn about human loading patterns as well.

Acknowledgments

The work reported here was supported by PHS grants DE11962 and DE08513. Shengyi Teng was responsible for the analysis of trabecular architecture and performed the early strain gage experiments. We also thank Kathy Rafferty, Scott Pedersen, Laurene Marks Wolf, In Choi and Trisha Emry for their participation in various aspects of these projects. The thoughtful comments of an anonymous reviewer helped us improve the manuscript.

References

Anapol, F., S.W. Herring (1989) Length-tension relationships of masseter and digastric muscles of miniature swine during ontogeny. J Exp Biol *143:* 1–16.

Bermejo, A., O. González, J.M. González (1993) The pig as an animal model for experimentation on the temporomandibular articular complex. Oral Surg Oral Med Oral Pathol *75:* 18–23.

Bertram, J.E.A., A.A. Biewener (1988) Bone curvature: Sacrificing strength for load predictability? J Theor Biol *131:* 75–92.

Crompton, A.W., W.L. Hylander (1986) Changes in mandibular function following the acquisition of a dentary-squamosal jaw articulation; in Hotton N, P.D. MacLean, J.J. Roth, E.C. Roth (eds): The Ecology and Biology of Mammal-like Reptiles. Washington, Smithsonian Institution Press, pp 263–282.

Dessem, D., R.E. Druzinsky (1992) Jaw-muscle activity in ferrets, *Mustela putorius furo.* J Morphol *213:* 275–286.

Goodship, A.E., L.E. Lanyon, H. McFie (1979) Functional adaptation of bone to increased stress. J Bone Jt Surg (Br) *61-A:* 539–546.

Greaves, W.S. (1980) The jaw lever system in ungulates: A new model. J Zool *184:* 271–285.

Herring, S.W. (1985) Morphological correlates of masticatory patterns in peccaries and pigs. J Mamm *66:* 603–617.

Herring, S.W. (1995) Animal models of temporomandibular disorders: how to choose; in Sessle B.J., P.S. Bryant, R.A. Dionne (eds): Temporomandibular Disorders and Related Pain Conditions. Seattle, IASP Press, pp 323–328.

Herring, S.W. (1998) How can animal models answer clinical questions?; in Carels C., G. Willems (eds): The Future of Orthodontics. Leuven, Leuven University Press, pp 89–96.

Herring, S.W., R.J. Mucci (1991) In vivo strain in cranial sutures: the zygomatic arch. J Morphol *207:* 225–239.

Herring, S.W., S. Teng (2000) Strain in the braincase and its sutures during function. Am J Phys Anthrop *112:* 575–593.

Hylander, W.L. (1975) The human mandible: Lever or link? Am J Phys Anthrop *43:* 227–242.

Hylander, W.L. (1979) An experimental analysis of temporomandibular joint reaction force in macaques. Am J Phys Anthrop *51:* 433–456.

Hylander, W.L., R. Bays (1979) An in vivo strain-gauge analysis of the squamosal-dentary joint reaction force during mastication and incisal biting in *Macaca mulatta* and *Macaca fascicularis.* Arch Oral Biol *24:* 689–697.

Lanyon, L.E. (1972) In vivo bone strain recorded from thoracic vertebrae of sheep. J Biomech *5:* 277–281.

Lanyon, L.E., W.G.J. Hampson, A.E. Goodship, J.S. Shah (1975) Bone deformation recorded in vivo from strain gauges attached to the human tibial shaft. Acta Orthop Scand *46:* 256–268.

Liu, Z.J., S.W. Herring (2000a) Bone surface strains and internal bony pressures at the jaw joint of the miniature pig during masticatory muscle contraction. Arch Oral Biol *45:* 95–112.

Liu, Z.J., S.W. Herring (2000b) Masticatory strains on osseous and ligamentous components of the jaw joint in miniature pigs. J Orofacial Pain *14:* 265–278.

Marks, L., S. Teng, J. Årtun, S. Herring (1997) Reaction strains on the condylar neck during mastication and maximum muscle stimulation in different condylar positions: An experimental study in the miniature pig. J Dent Res *76:* 1412–1420.

Martin, R.B., D.B. Burr, N.A. Sharkey (1998) Skeletal Tissue Mechanics. New York, Springer.

Odgaard, A. (1997) Three-dimensional methods for quantification of cancellous bone architecture. Bone *20:* 315–328.

Rafferty, K.L., S.W. Herring, F. Artese (2000) Three-dimensional loading and growth of the zygomatic arch. J Exptl Biol *203:* 2093–3004.

Sindelar, B.J., S.P. Evanko, T. Alonzo, S.W. Herring, T. Wight (2000) Effects of intraoral splint wear on proteoglycans in the temporomandibular joint disc. Arch Biochem Biophys *379:* 64–70.

Ström, D., S. Holm, E. Clemensson, T. Haraldson, G.E. Carlsson (1986) Gross anatomy of the mandibular joint and masticatory muscles in the domestic pig *(Sus scrofa).* Arch Oral Biol *31:* 763–768.

Swartz, S.M. (1991) Strain analysis as a tool for functional morphology. Am Zool *31:* 655–669.

Teng, S., I.W. Choi, S.W. Herring, J.M. Rensberger (1997) Stereological analysis of bone architecture in the pig zygomatic arch. Anat Rec *248:* 205–213.

Teng, S., S.W. Herring (1995) A stereological study of trabecular architecture in the mandibular condyle of the pig. Arch Oral Biol *40:* 299–310.

Teng, S., S.W. Herring (1996) Anatomical and directional variation in the mechanical properties of the mandibular condyle in pigs. J Dent Res *75:* 1842–1850.

Throckmorton, G.S., G.J. Groshan, S.B. Boyd (1990) Muscle activity patterns and control of temporomandibular joint loads. J Prosth Dent *63:* 685–695.

Wainwright, S.A. (1988) Axis and Circumference. Cambridge, Harvard.

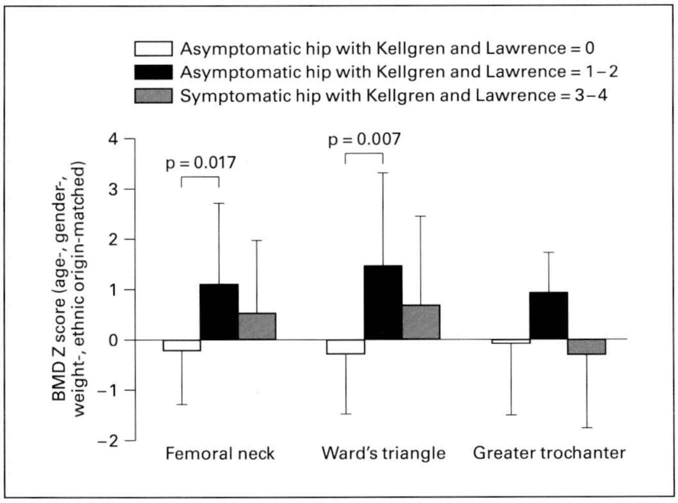

Fig. 2. Hip joints with early asymptomatic degeneration had increased proximal femoral BMD as compared to those with no radiographic evidence of hip degeneration. Modified from Bruno et al. [1999].

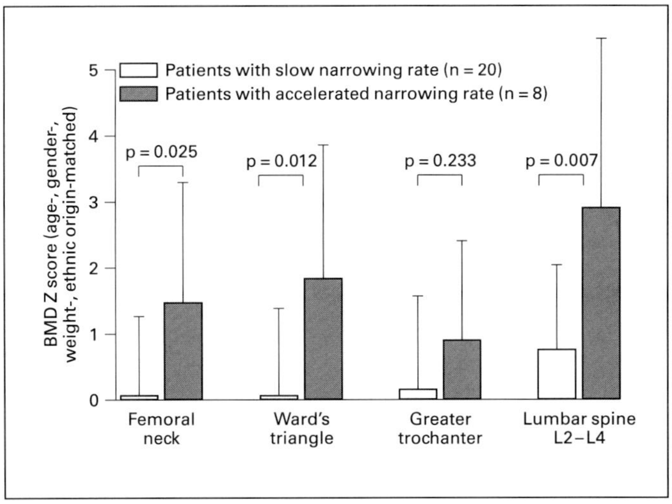

Fig. 3. The proximal femoral and lumbar BMD were greater in subjects with a subsequent accelerated narrowing rate as compared to those with a slow narrowing rate.

apparent late decrease in BMD could be related to pain and decreased loading of the joint as described in more detail, below.

Elevated BMD and a Subsequent Accelerated Joint Space Narrowing Rate

In another study, twenty-eight subjects who underwent THR for OA and who had an asymptomatic contralateral hip had their proximal femur on the asymptomatic contralateral side and lumbar spine scanned by DXA [Goker et al., 2000b]. The joint space narrowing rate in the asymptomatic hip was determined by serial longitudinal quantification of the joint space width. The minimal detectable change in joint space width was determined to be 0.07 mm [Goker et al., 2000b].

Eight subjects were classified as having an accelerated rate (>0.2 mm/year) and 20 subjects were classified as having a slow rate (≤0.2 mm/year). A 2-way analysis of variance (ANOVA) indicated that joint space narrowing rate category (slow or accelerated) but not modified KL grade, accounted for a significant proportion of the variance in the BMD data. Subjects with a subsequent accelerated narrowing rate had higher initial BMD than subjects with a slow narrowing rate (fig. 3). While this finding may appear to conflict with the previous study, it actually indicates that the rate of joint space narrowing and not the modified KL grade accounts for more of the variation in BMD. Although the baseline BMD was higher in those with an accelerated narrowing rate, the BMD values did not change significantly in either group during the two year course of the study. Thus, the presence of elevated BMD in both the involved and distant sites in subjects who subsequently had an accelerated joint space narrowing rate suggests that bone may be involved in the early pathogenesis of OA.

Gait Adaptations and Hip OA

In examining the role of bone in disease progression, it is critical to consider the femur's mechanical environment. Subjects with end-stage hip OA walk with significantly reduced moments and hip range of motion as compared to normal subjects [Hurwitz et al., 1997]. In a recent study, joint motion, moments and intersegmental forces were calculated for 19 subjects with unilateral hip OA and 19 normal subjects with a similar age distribution. The subjects with hip OA walked with a decreased dynamic hip range of motion (17 ± 4°) compared to normal subjects (29 ± 7°, $p < 0.001$). The subjects with hip OA walked with significantly lower than normal extension, adduction and internal and external rotation moments in their affected hips (fig. 4). The extension moment was inversely correlated with pain ($R = -0.78$, $p < 0.001$), suggesting that decreased muscle force in the hip flexors may be a mechanism to adapt to pain.

Another recent study has shown that some gait characteristics associated with end-stage hip OA are associated with early radiographic signs of asymptomatic hip degeneration [Hurwitz et al., 1999]. Fifteen subjects scheduled

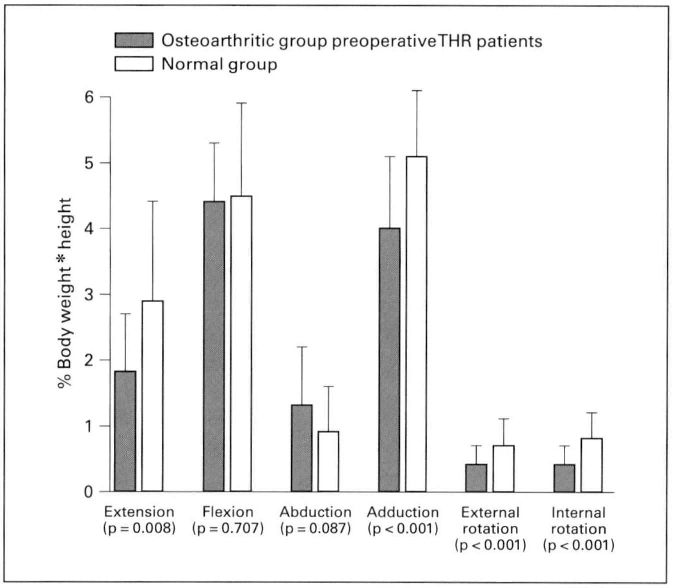

Fig. 4. The subjects with endstage hip OA had significantly decreased extension, adduction and internal and external rotations moments as compared to normal subjects.

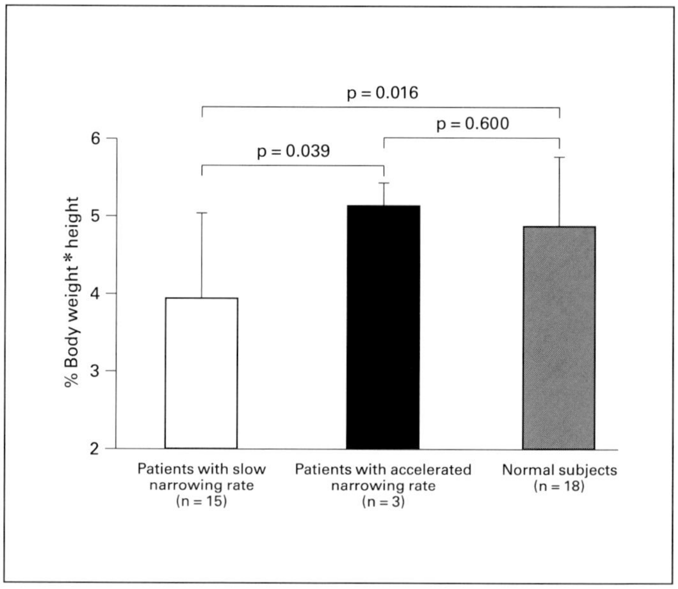

Fig. 5. The hip adduction moment was significantly greater in subjects with an accelerated narrowing rate than those subjects with a slow narrowing rate.

for unilateral THR for OA with no other significant lower extremity pathology were tested with gait analysis just prior to surgery. Thirteen of the subjects were also retested one year postoperatively. Subjects were stratified into two groups based on the modified KL grade [Felson et al., 1995] of the asymptomatic hip. One group consisted of 3 subjects without radiographic evidence of contralateral hip degeneration (modified KL grade of 0) and the other group consisted of 12 subjects with radiographic evidence of hip degeneration (modified KL grades of 1, 2 or 3). To determine if the hip biomechanics during gait of the asymptomatic side of either group were similar to those with end-stage hip OA, the preoperative THR side was also tested along with 21 normal subjects.

The asymptomatic hips with radiographic changes (modified KL grades of 1–3) had a significantly decreased peak intersegmental hip fore force and internal rotation moment than the asymptomatic hips with no radiographic changes (modified KL grade of 0) ($p < 0.024$). While the gait changes on the asymptomatic side described above were associated with the presence of radiographic hip degeneration, an increased flexion moment ($p = 0.036$) and a decreased adduction moment ($p = 0.013$) as compared to normal subjects occurred on the asymptomatic side regardless of the radiographic status. The gait adaptations on the contralateral side present preoperatively persisted postoperatively.

Thus, both before and after THR, subjects with unilateral end-stage hip OA load their contralateral hip joint differently from normal. These alterations in loading may have implications with regard to the rate of progression or pathogenesis of hip degeneration in subjects beginning to develop bilateral degeneration.

Increased Joint Loading and a Subsequent Accelerated Narrowing Rate

The gait of the contralateral side of 18 subjects scheduled for a unilateral THR for primary OA was tested preoperatively in another study [Lowinger et al., 2000]. Selection criteria included absence of other significant lower extremity pathology, a modified KL grade [Felson et al., 1995] or 2 or less and an initial joint space width of at least 1 mm on the contralateral side. The joint space narrowing rate on the contralateral side was determined from at least 3 radiographs taken over a minimum of the next three years with the initial radiograph taken perioperatively. Three subjects had an accelerated narrowing rate (>0.2 mm/year) and 15 subjects, a slow narrowing rate (≤0.2 mm/year). The subjects with an accelerated narrowing rate had a significantly greater preoperative peak adduction moment than the subjects with a slow narrowing rate (p 0.039; fig. 5). The peak hip adduction moment is a major determinant of the peak hip contact force [Foucher et al., 1999]. Subjects with an accelerated narrowing rate had a normal adduction moment ($p = 0.600$) while subjects with a slow narrowing rate had a lower than normal peak hip adduction moment ($p = 0.016$). This suggests gait adaptations leading to reduced joint loads may 'protect' the joint and lead to a slower joint narrowing rate.

Interrelationship between Loading and BMD

Load history among subjects with end-stage hip OA, as determined by the calculation of the hip moments during walking, influenced the distribution of proximal femoral BMD [Hurwitz et al., 1998a]. Gait analysis and DXA scans of the proximal femur were acquired for 25 candidates for unilateral THR, all with a diagnosis of end-stage hip OA. The greater trochanter BMD Z score on the affected side was significantly correlated with the external rotation moment ($R = 0.648$, $p < 0.001$), the dynamic hip range of motion ($R = 0.50$, $p = 0.011$) and the adduction moment ($R = 0.43$, $p = 0.032$) while the femoral neck BMD Z score was significantly correlated with the adduction moment ($R = 0.54$, $p = 0.005$). More subjects had decreased greater trochanter BMD on the end-stage OA side (76%) than would be expected for a normal population ($p = 0.015$) while more subjects had increased femoral neck BMD on the end-stage OA side (72%) than would be expected for a normal population ($p = 0.046$). Thus, in end-stage OA there was a correlation between BMD and loading at a site of increased BMD (femoral neck) and at a site of decreased BMD (greater trochanter).

The abductors are the primary muscles that balance the adduction moment. They insert on the greater trochanter so that a reduced adduction moment may reflect reduced forces in the greater trochanter and may result in bone loss in this region. Moreover, the anterior fibers of the gluteus medius and minimus muscles are primary internal rotators [Spence and Mason, 1979; Moore, 1985; Kapandji, 1987; Mansour and Pereira, 1987] so that the decreased external rotation moment during early stance may also be reflective of decreased abductor muscle forces. The significant correlation between the femoral neck and Ward's triangle BMD and the adduction moment is likely due to a decreased contact force and bending moment in the femoral neck resulting from a decreased adduction moment. While there may have been a systemic increase in the BMD at these two sites, there is also an additional influence of loading. In particular, the between subject variation in the BMD was correlated with the between subject variation in the adduction moment.

This study provides evidence that load history as determined by calculation of the hip moments during level walking, influences the regional distribution of proximal femoral BMD in an end-stage hip OA population.

Summary

Our data indicate that some subjects with a history of unilateral end-stage hip OA may also have alterations in BMD and gait adaptations on their asymptomatic contralateral side that are associated with early radiographic hip degeneration. Moreover, a subset of these subjects with a THR may have an accelerated joint space narrowing rate on their contralateral side. These subjects with accelerated joint space narrowing rates had higher BMD and higher adduction moments during gait than those subjects with slower joint space narrowing rates. Based on cross-sectional data, it has also been shown that among subjects with end-stage hip OA, proximal femoral BMD [Bruno et al., 1999; Hurwitz et al., 1998a] and gait [Hurwitz et al., 1997] are different from normal and that proximal femoral BMD is related to hip joint loads during walking [Hurwitz et al., 1998a]. Thus, while decreases in hip joint loading during gait and changes in the proximal femoral BMD patterns are two characteristics of end-stage hip OA, they are interrelated. The studies on the association between early radiographic hip degeneration and gait or BMD and joint space narrowing rate were each done on separate subject groups and in some cases the sample sizes were relatively small. It cannot be determined from these data if the increased BMD associated with the early radiographic hip degeneration or subsequent accelerated narrowing rate is influenced by the hip joint loading. Thus, the combined ability that the dynamic hip joint loads during gait and the proximal femoral BMD have in explaining the variance in the joint space narrowing rate has yet to be determined and is the subject of an ongoing prospective investigation at our institution.

Acknowledgements

Whitaker grant, NIH SCOR AR39239, NIH AR46225, Depuy grant.

References

Akmatsu, Y., T. Koshino, T. Saito, J. Wada (1997) Changes in osteosclerosis of the osteoarthritic knee after high tibial osteotomy. Clin Orthop Rel Res *334:* 207–214.

Andersson, J.J., D.T. Felson (1988) Factors associated with osteoarthritis of the knee in the first National Health and Nutrition Examination Survey (NHANESI). Evidence for an association with overweight, race and physical demands of work. Am J Epidemiol *128:* 179–189.

Andriacchi, T.P., R.N. Natarajan, D.E. Hurwitz (1997) Musculoskeletal dynamic locomotion and clinical applications; in Mow V.C., W.C. Hayes (eds): Basic Orthopaedic Biomechanics, ed 2. New York, Raven Press, pp 37–69.

Boyde, A., S.J. Jones, J. Aerssens, J. Dequeker (1995) Mineral density quantitation of the human cortical iliac crest by backscattered electron image analysis: Variations with age, sex, and degree of osteoarthritis. Bone *16:* 619–627.

Bruno, R.J., A.P. Sauer, A.G. Rosenberg, J. Block, D.R. Sumner (1999) The pattern of bone mineral density in the proximal femur and radiographic signs of early joint degeneration. J Rheum *26:* 636–640.

Bryan, J.M., D.R. Sumner, D.E. Hurwitz, G.S. Tomkins, T.P. Andriacchi, J.O. Galante (1996) Altered load history affects periprosthetic bone loss following cementless total hip arthroplasty. J Orthop Res *14:* 762–768.

Burger, H., P.L.A. van Daele, E. Odding, H.A. Valkenburg, A. Hofman, D.E. Grobbee, H.E. Schutte, J.C. Birkenhager, H.A.P. Pols (1996) Association of radiographically evident osteoarthritis with higher bone mineral density and increased bone loss with age. Arthritis Rheum *39:* 81–86.

Burr, D.B., R.B. Martin (1992) Mechanisms of bone adaptation to the mechanical environment. Triangle *31:* 59–76.

Burr, D.B., M.B. Schaffler (1997) The involvement of subchondral mineralized tissues in osteoarthritis: Quantitative microscopic evidence. Microsc Res Techn *37:* 343–357.

Carter, D.R., T.E. Orr, D.P. Fyhrie (1989) Relationships between loading history and femoral bone architecture. J Biomech *22:* 231–244.

Christensen, P., J. Kjaer, F. Melsen, H.E. Nielsen, O. Snepper, P.V. Vang (1982) The subchondral bone of the proximal tibial epiphysis in osteoarthritis of the knee. Acta Orthop Scand *53:* 889–895.

Cooper, C., P.L. Cook, C. Osmond, L. Fisher, M.I.D. Cawley (1991) Osteoarthritis of the hip and osteoporosis of the proximal femur. Ann Rheum Dis *50:* 540–542.

Croft, P., D. Coggon, M. Cruddas et al (1992) Osteoarthritis of the hip: As an occupational disease in farmers. BMJ *304:* 1269–1272.

Dequeker, J., J. Aerssens (1993a) Bone mineral density and osteoarthritis. Ann Rheum Dis *52:* 316.

Dequeker, J., O. Johnell (1993b) Osteoarthritis protects against femoral neck fracture: the MEDOS study experience. Bone *14:* S51–S56.

Dequeker, J., S. Mohan, R.D. Finkelman, J. Aerssens, D.J. Baylink (1993) Generalized osteoarthritis associated with increased insulin-like growth factor types I and II and transforming growth factor beta in cortical bone from the iliac crest: Possible mechanism of increased bone density and protection against osteoporosis. Arthritis Rheum *36:* 1702–1708.

Dequeker, J., L. Mokassa, J. Aerssens (1995) Bone density and osteoarthritis. J Rheum *22S:* 98–100.

Dequeker, J., R. Westhovens (1994) Distinction between initiation and progression of the osteoarthritis process. Ann Rheum Dis *53:* 356.

Dougados, M., A. Gueguen, M. Nguyen, L. Berdah, M. Lesquesne, B. Mazières, E. Vignon (1999) Requirement for total hip arthroplasty: an outcome measure of hip osteoarthritis? J Rheum *26:* 855–861.

Doughan, A.M., B. Goker, T.J. Schnitzer, L. Kull, J.A. Block (1997) Time course of contralateral total hip arthroplasty after hip replacement for osteoarthritis. Trans ORS *22:* 283.

Fazzalari, N.L. (1993) Trabecular microfracture. Calcif Tissue Int *53:* S143–S147.

Fazzalari, N.L., I.H. Parkinson (1997) Fractal properties of subchondral cancellous bone in severe osteoarthritis of the hip. J Bone Miner Res *12:* 632–640.

Felson, D.T., M.T. Hannan, A. Naimark et al (1991) Occupational physical demands, knee bending, and knee osteoarthritis: Results from the Framingham Study. J Rheumatol *118:* 1587–1592.

Felson, D.T. (1993) The course of osteoarthritis and factors that affect it. Rheum Dis Clin North Am *19:* 607–615.

Felson, D.T., Y. Zhang, M. Hannan, A. Naimark, B.N. Weissman, P. Aliabadi, P. Levy (1995) The incidence and natural history of knee osteoarthritis in the elderly: The Framingham Osteoarthritis study. Arthritis Rheum *38:* 1500–1505.

Felts, W., E. Yelin (1989) The economic impact of the rheumatic diseases in the United States. J Rheumatol *16:* 867–884.

Fischer, K.J., C.R. Jacobs, M.E. Levenston, D.R. Carter (1996) Different loads can produce similar bone density distributions. Bone *19:* 127–135.

Flygare, L., H. Hosoki, A. Petersson, M. Rohlin, S. Akerman (1997) Bone volume in human temporomandibular autopsy joints with and without erosive changes. Acta Odontol Scand *55:* 167–172.

Foss, M.V.L., P.D. Byers (1972) Bone density, osteoarthritis of the hip, and fracture of the upper end of the femur. Ann Rheum Dis *31:* 259–264.

Foucher, K.C., D.E. Hurwitz, T.P. Andriacchi (1999) Gait Adaptations in Postoperative Total Hip Replacement Patients Are Associated with Reduced Hip Contact Forces. San Diego, American Society of Biomechanics, pp 134–135.

Frost, H.M. (1990a) Skeletal structural adaptations to mechanical usage (SATMU). 1. Redefining Wolff's law: The bone modeling problem. Anat Rec *226:* 403–413.

Frost, H.M. (1990b) Skeletal structural adaptations to mechanical usage (SATMU). 2. Redefining Wolff's law: The remodeling problem. Anat Rec *226:* 414–422.

Goker, B., A. Doughan, T.J. Schnitzer, J.A. Block (2000a) Quantification of progressive joint space narrowing in osteoarthritis of the hip: Longitudinal analysis of the contralateral hip after total hip arthroplasty. J Arthr Rheum *43:* 988–994.

Goker, B., D.R. Sumner, D.E. Hurwitz, J.A. Block (2000b) Bone mineral density varies as a function of the joint space narrowing rate in the hip. J Rheumatol *27:* 735–738.

Gotfredsen, A., B.J. Riis, C. Christiansen, P. Rodbro (1990) Does a single local absorptiometric bone measurement indicate the overall skeletal status? Implications for osteoporosis and osteoarthritis of the hip. Clin Rheumatol *9:* 193–203.

Goldberg, V., K. Kuettner (eds) (1995) Osteoarthritic Disorders: Workshop, Monterey, California, April 1994. Rosemont, American Academy of Orthopaedic Surgeons, pp xxii–xxiii.

Hamerman, D., E.R. Stanley (1996) Implications of increased bone density in osteoarthritis. J Bone Miner Res *11:* 1205–1208.

Hordon, L.D., V. Wright, M.A. Smith (1992) Bone mass in osteoarthritis. Ann Rheum Dis *51:* 823–825.

Huiskes, R., J.D. Janssen, T.J. Slooff (1981) A detailed comparison of experimental and theoretical stress-analyses of a human femur; in Cowin S.C. (ed): Mechanical Properties of Bone. New York, American Society of Mechanical Engineering, p 211.

Hvid, I. (1988) Trabecular bone strength at the knee. Clin Orthop Rel Res *227:* 210–221.

Hvid, I., S.L. Hansen (1985) Trabecular bone strength patterns at the proximal tibial epiphysis. J Orthop Res *3:* 464–472.

Hurwitz, D.E., K.C. Foucher, D.R. Sumner, T.P. Andriacchi, A.G. Rosenberg, J.O. Galante (1998a) Hip motion and moment during gait relate directly to proximal femoral bone mineral density in patients with hip osteoarthritis. J Biomech *31:* 919–926.

Hurwitz, D.E., C.H. Hulet, T.P. Andriacchi, A.G. Rosenberg, J.O. Galante (1997) Gait compensations in patients with hip osteoarthritis and their relationship to pain and passive hip motion. JOR *15:* 629–635.

Hurwitz, D.E., D.R. Sumner, T.P. Andriacchi, D.A. Sugar (1998b) Dynamic knee loads during gait predict proximal tibial bone distribution. J Biomech *31:* 423–430.

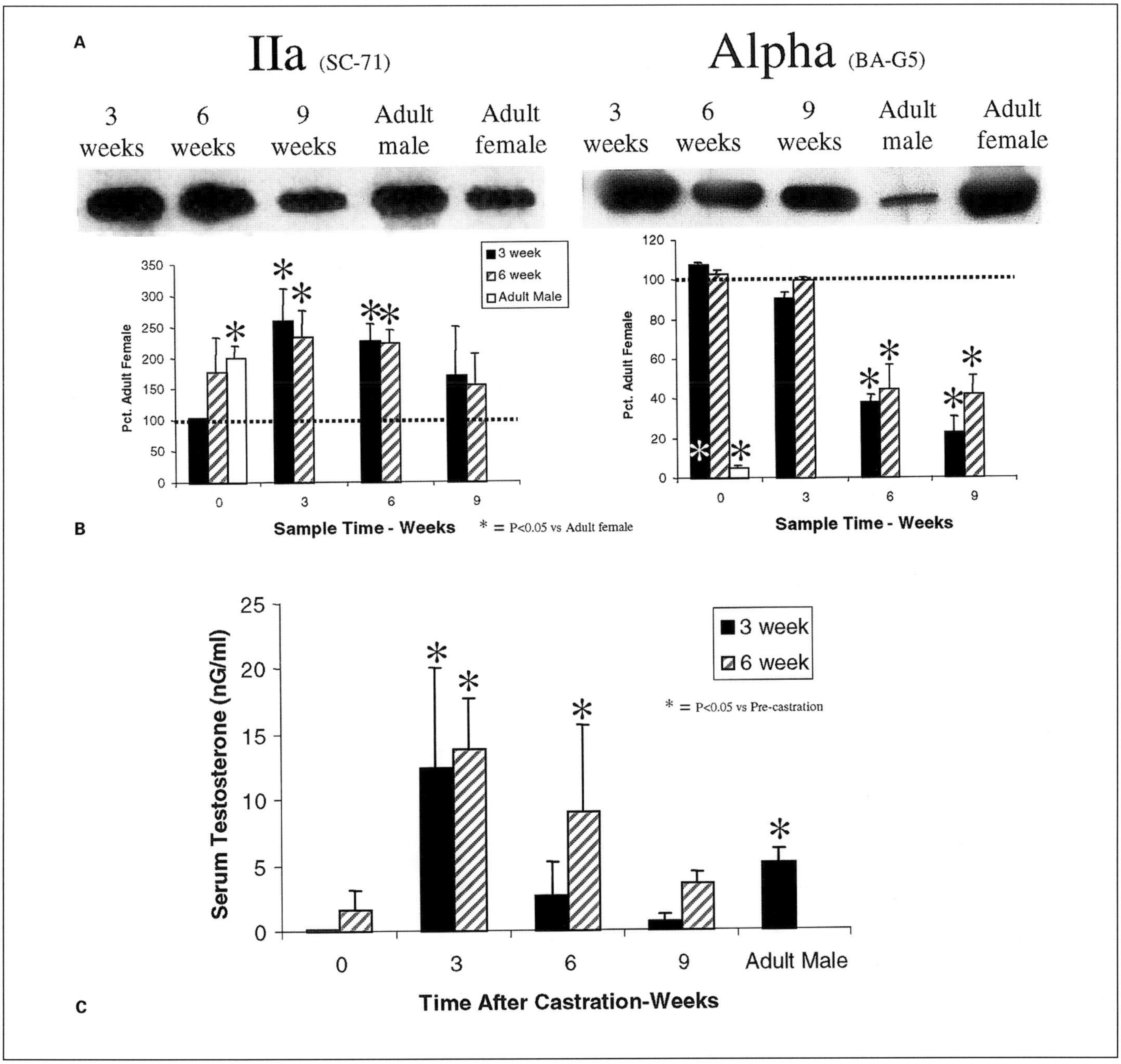

Fig. 1. A Representative immunoblots for the IIa (left) and cardiac alpha (right)-MyHC isoforms. Samples of equal protein content were loaded into adjacent lanes of an SDS-PAGE gel consisting of an 8% separating gel and a 4% stacking gel and electrophoresed at room temperature for 1 h. After transfer to membranes, they were probed either with antibody SC-71 for the IIa MyHC isoform, or antibody BA-G5 for the cardiac alpha-MyHC isoform. Immunoreactivity was detected using ECL. Samples used in these blots were from biopsies of the masseter muscles of an animal castrated as a young adult and given testosterone for 6 weeks. Biopsies were made at 3, 6 and 9 weeks after castration. In these blots and all others used in this series, samples from the masseter of an adult male and an adult female were run on the same gel. **B** Results from densitometric analyses of immunoblots. Each band on each blot was scanned and the intensity of immunoreactivity was measured three times. The average of these measures was then expressed as a percentage of the average for the adult female and used to compute a mean (±SEM) for the two samples in each series. These values at different times after castration are then plotted in the graphs. The dashed lines indicate the values of 100% of the adult female. * Values that are significantly ($p < 0.05$) different from precastration values. **C** Results of analysis of serum testosterone measurements in these animals. Each bar reflects the mean (±SEM) testosterone level expressed in nG/ml. Adult male values are the average measured from samples of serum of 3 animals. + Significant ($p < 0.05$) differences from precastration levels.

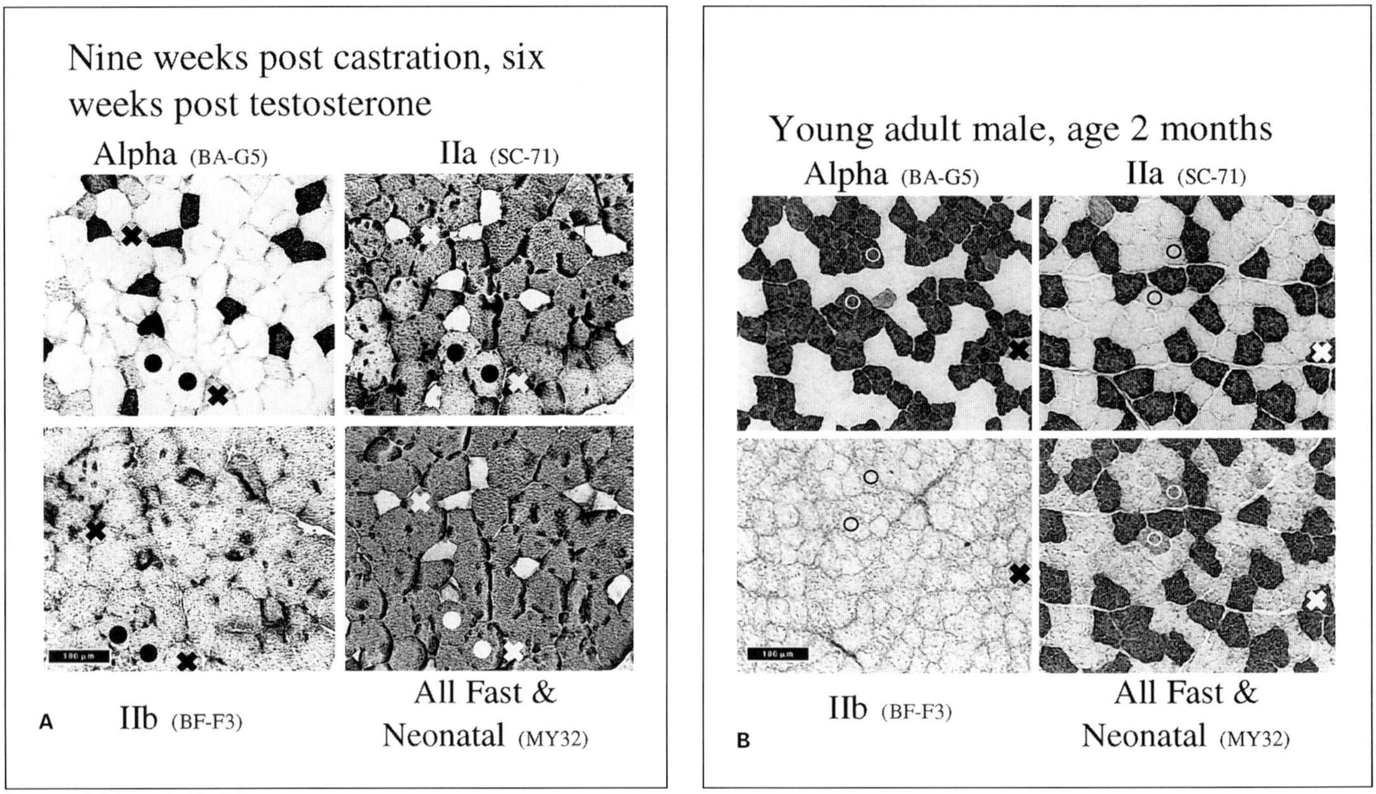

Fig. 2. Histological analyses of masseter muscle samples. The four images in each panel are taken from sequential serial cryostat sections of biopsies from the masseter muscle of a male rabbit. **A** Images are from sections of a biopsy taken 9 weeks after the animal had been castrated and had been given testosterone for 3 weeks. **B** Images are from sections of a biopsy taken at the time of castration. Each of the sections used in the montage in each panel was stained using a monoclonal antibody specific to a different MyHC isoform. The name of the antibody used and its specificity are shown next to each panel. The images obtained were aligned to enable the examination of the same fibers in different sections. Of particular interest are fibers staining weakly with antibody BA-G5 and strongly with antibody SC-71 (marked with an 'X') in **A**) (alpha/slow/IIa fibers), and fibers staining weakly with antibody SC-71 but reacting strongly with antibody MY32. These fibers are suspected of containing both the IIa and type IIx MyHC isoforms. Representatives are indicated by filled circles (●) in **A**. Note that fibers of these phenotypes are not found in **B**. **B** Some fibers staining with antibody MY32 and the antibody to the cardiac alpha MyHC isoform, but not with antibodies to the IIa or IIb isoforms. These fibers are suspected of containing the cardiac alpha (and slow) MyHC isoform as well as the neonatal MyHC isoform. Representatives are indicated by open circles (○) in **B**. Note that fibers of these phenotypes are not found in **A**.

and only slightly more frequently in young adult males [Eason et al., 2000b].

Several of the larger fibers in muscles from testosterone treated animals react weakly with the antibody to the IIa MyHC isoform, not at all with the IIb antibody, but strongly with antibody MY32, which recognizes all type II and the neonatal MyHC isoforms (fig. 2A, closed circles). Such a combination of immunoreactivity is consistent with these fibers containing both the IIa and IIx (IId) MyHC isoforms. Fibers of this phenotype were found in samples of muscles from testosterone treated animals at all ages studied (data not shown). Fibers with this staining pattern were not encountered in our studies of muscles from untreated animals (fig. 2B) [English et al., 1999].

In muscles from untreated young adult male rabbits, we found some fibers that reacted both to antibody MY32 (all fast and neonatal) and to antibodies to the slow and cardiac alpha MyHC isoforms, but not with antibodies to the IIa or to the IIb MyHC isoforms (fig. 2B, open circles). We believe that these fibers contain the slow, alpha, and neonatal MyHC isoforms, since Bredman et al. [1992] have described fibers of this phenotype in animals of this age. We did not encounter these fibers in any muscles from testosterone-treated animals.

Discussion

The main finding of this study is that exposing young adult rabbits to testosterone for as little as three weeks induces a MyHC isoform switch that persists well beyond the exposure to the hormone. The rabbit masseter is sexually dimorphic with respect to the proportions of muscle fibers of different phenotypes [English et al., 1999]. These sex differences arise under the influence of testosterone during postnatal development, and are expressed as a MyHC isoform switch from slow/alpha to IIa [d'Albis et al., 1993; Eason et al., 2000b]. Castration of adult rabbits does not alter these differences in phenotype proportions, indicating that the isoform switch is essentially permanent [Eason et al., 2000b]. In this study, brief exposure to testosterone induced a qualitatively similar isoform switch. Based on our analysis of serum testosterone, we assume that the much-elevated levels found during treatment will have dropped precipitously in these castrated animals when the exogenous hormone was discontinued. At the time of final examination, testosterone levels have been reduced for either 3 or 6 weeks.

Myosin heavy chain isoform switches are the most widely known form of muscle plasticity. There are five known MyHC isoforms found in adult mammalian limb and jaw muscles, and based on available evidence [Schiaffino and Reggiani, 1996] fibers can switch from expressing one to another according to a relatively rigid format described by the following plan:

$$I/\alpha \leftrightarrows IIa \leftrightarrows IIx \leftrightarrows IIb.$$

During normal postnatal development in young adult male rabbits, some fibers stop expressing the slow (type I) and cardiac alpha isoforms and begin to express the IIa isoform [Eason et al., 2000b]. In this study, brief exposure to testosterone in young adult males resulted in a decrease in the cardiac alpha MyHC isoform and an increase in the IIa MyHC isoform. This MyHC isoform switch might be expected if such exposure to testosterone were sufficient to explain the normal development of the adult male proportions of fibers of different phenotypes in the masseter. Our finding that some fibers contain both the cardiac alpha and IIa MyHC isoforms in testosterone treated animals but not in normal animals might be interpreted as instances of fibers in the process of this isoform switch.

However, because we found that the amount of the IIa isoform actually decreases after its initial increase, and because we found several large fibers that are only weakly immunoreactive for the IIa MyHC isoform, we suspect that our hormone treatments did more than mimic normal development. We interpret these findings as evidence that the hormone treatment not only caused some fibers to switch to IIa from slow/alpha but other fibers were induced to switch from containing only the IIa MyHC isoform to contain both IIa and IIx.

There is currently no antibody that recognizes only the IIa MyHC isoform, so that we cannot be absolutely certain of identification of this isoform at the protein level. In adult male rabbits, we have found little evidence for the presence of the IIx MyHC isoform in the masseter muscle [English et al., 1999], although Pette's group have reported finding the mRNA for this isoform in the rabbit masseter [Aigner et al., 1993]. We [English et al., 1999] and others [Aigner et al., 1993] have found no evidence for the IIb MyHC isoform in the rabbit masseter. Our hormone treatment resulted in the appearance of large fibers with weak immunoreactivity to the IIa MyHC isoform (antibody SC-71) and intense immunoreactivity to an antibody recognizing all type II isoforms and the neonatal MyHC isoform (MY32). Although we cannot rule out the re-appearance of the neonatal MyHC isoform, we contend that this observation is most compatible with the induction of the IIx gene in these fibers. It is not clear why such a change occurs. It is not found during normal development. We can only speculate that the supraphysiologic doses of testosterone we administered induced this switch.

Changes in MyHC isoform content induced by testosterone treatment did not occur simultaneously, at least at the protein level, but they did persist beyond the cessation of the treatment. The relative amount of the cardiac alpha-MyHC isoform decreased after testosterone treatment, and this decrease persisted well after serum testosterone levels had returned to precastration levels. Although the proportions of the IIa MyHC isoform returned to pre-castration values after the removal of hormone, this change does not mark a return to precastration conditions. It is more likely to reflect the quantitative decrease of the IIa MyHC isoform and the presence of the IIx isoform observed in some fibers using histological methods. It will be important in future studies to include even longer survival periods to be able to assess whether hormone-induced changes in MyHC isoform expression are irreversible, as they are during normal rabbit development [Eason et al., 2000b].

The control of MyHC isoform expression is largely believed to reside in the motoneurons innervating muscle fibers [Pette and Staron, 1997]. In particular, the activity pattern of the neuron is thought to promote either a slow (or slow/alpha) phenotype or fast (type II) phenotype in the muscle fibers innervated [Pette and Staron, 1997]. This *neurogenic* perspective is based largely on the results of cross-reinnervation and chronic electrical stimulation experiments, and more recently on the hypothesis that the mechanism of such neurogenic regulation of muscle fiber protein expression involves calcium signaling through the calcium/calmodulin dependent phosphatase, calcineurin [Chin et al., 1998]. Alternatively, hormones are known to exert an effect on contractile protein expression, especially on muscles of mastication [Hanzlikova and Gutmann, 1974; Inoue et al., 1994] and their effect is generally considered direct or *myogenic*. It is not known whether the effects of testosterone such as those described above are myogenic, neurogenic, or both. In the present study we described robust effects of testosterone exposure that could be used as part of a paradigm designed to evaluate these different models. In studies of the effects of thyroid hormone in mediating MyHC isoform switching in limb muscles, Baldwin's group [Adams et al., 1999] concluded that both neurogenic and myogenic factors are involved.

The functional consequences of the sex differences in muscle fiber phenotype proportions are not yet known. Based on the intrinsic rates of shortening and specific tension reported for fibers of the alpha/slow and IIa phenotypes [Walters et al., 1991; Eldred et al., 1993; Fukunaga et al., 1996] one might predict that the masseter muscles of adult male rabbits would produce greater forces more rapidly than the same muscles of females. However, such a consideration might be too simplistic. Fibers of the IIa phenotype are, on average, nearly 50% larger in females than fibers of the same phenotype in males, and they are nearly three times larger than fibers of the alpha/slow phenotype of either sex [English et al., 1999]. Assuming that motor units in the rabbit masseter are recruited in an orderly fashion by size [Cope and Sokoloff, 1999], one might expect that at low to moderate levels of activation, when only slow/alpha-containing motor units might be active, the forces produced by the masseter in males and females might be comparable. At slightly higher levels of activation, males, but not females, will recruit motor units containing IIa fibers, and they might be expected to produce larger forces more rapidly. Because IIa fibers are so much larger in females, once motor units containing them are recruited, their effect will be dominant and the forces produced by the masseter muscles of females might be expected to be greater than that of males. We do not yet know whether such sex differences in muscle function at high levels of motor unit recruitment exist, nor do we know whether such differences could account for some or all of the sex differences in chronic musculoskeletal pain in the head and neck reported clinically.

Acknowledgements

This work was supported by grant DE11536 from the USPHS. Thanks to Dr. Charles Widmer for reading an earlier draft of the manuscript.

References

Adams, G.R., S.A. McCue, M. Zeng, K.M. Baldwin (1999) Time course of myosin heavy chain transitions in neonatal rats: Importance of innervation and thyroid state. Am J Physiol Reg Integr Comp Physiol *276:* R954–R961.

Aigner, S., B. Gohlsch, N. Hamalainen, R.S. Staron, A. Uber, U. Wehrle, D. Pette (1993) Fast myosin heavy chain diversity in skeletal muscles of the rabbit: Heavy chain IId, not IIb predominates. Eur J Biochem *211:* 367–372.

Bredman, J.J., W.A. Weijs, H.A. Korfage, P. Brugman, A.F. Moorman (1992) Myosin heavy chain expression in rabbit masseter muscle during postnatal development. J Anat *180:* 263–274.

Chin, E.R., E.N. Olson, J.A. Richardson, Q. Yang, C. Humphries, J.M. Shelton, H. Wu, W. Zhu, R. Bassel-Duby, R.S. Williams (1998) A calcineurin-dependent transcriptional pathway controls skeletal muscle fiber type. Genes Dev *12:* 2499–2509.

Cope, T.C., A.J. Sokoloff (1999) Orderly recruitment among motoneurons supplying different muscles. J Physiol Paris *93:* 81–85.

d'Albis, A., R. Couteaux, C. Janmot, J.C. Mira (1993) Opposite regulations by androgenic and thyroid hormones of V1 myosin expression in the two types of rabbit striated muscle: Skeletal and cardiac. Febs Lett *318:* 53–56.

Eason, J., G. Schwartz, G. Pavlath, A. English (2000a) Sexually dimorphic expression of myosin heavy chain isoforms in adult mouse masseter muscles. J Appl Physiol *89:* 251–258.

Eason, J., M.G. Schwartz, K.A. Shirley, A.W. English (2000b) Investigation of sexual dimorphism in the rabbit masseter muscle showing different effects of androgen deprivation in adult and young adult animals. Arch Oral Biol *45:* 683–690.

Eldred, E., A. Garfinkel, E.S. Hsu, M. Ounjian, R.R. Roy, V.R. Edgerton (1993) The physiological cross-sectional area of motor units in the cat tibialis anterior. Anat Rec *235:* 381–389.

English, A., J. Eason, G. Schwartz, A. Shirley (1999) Sexual dimorphism in the rabbit masseter muscle: Myosin heavy chain composition of neuromuscular compartments. Cells Tissues Organs *164:* 179–191.

English, A.W., J. Eason, M. Pol, G. Schwartz, A. Shirley (1998) Different phenotypes among slow/beta myosin heavy chain-containing fibers of rabbit masseter muscle: A novel type of diversity in adult muscle. J Mus Res Cell Motil *19:* 525–535.

English, A.W., S.L. Wolf, R.L. Segal (1993) Compartmentalization of muscles and their motor nuclei: The partitioning hypothesis. Phys Ther *73:* 857–867.

Fukunaga, T., R.R. Roy, F.G. Shellock, J.A. Hodgson, V.R. Edgerton (1996) Specific tension of human plantar flexors and dorsiflexors. J Appl Physiol *80:* 158–165.

Gutmann, E., V. Hanzlikova, Z. Lojda (1970) Effect of androgens on histochemical fibre type: Differentiation in the temporal muscle of the guinea pig. Histochemie *24:* 287–291.

Hanzlikova, V., E. Gutmann (1974) The absence of androgen-sensitivity in the grafted soleus muscle innervated by the pudendal nerve. Cell Tiss Res *154:* 121–129.

Inoue, K., S. Yamasaki, T. Fushiki, Y. Okada, E. Sugimoto (1994) Androgen receptor antagonist suppresses exercise-induced hypertrophy of skeletal muscle. Eur J Appl Physiol Occup Physiol *69:* 88–91.

Kelly, A., G. Lyons, B. Gambki, N. Rubinstein (1985) Influences of testosterone on contractile proteins of the guinea pig temporalis muscle. Adv Exp Med Biol *182:* 155–168.

Maxwell, L.C., D.C. Carlson, J.A. McNamara, J.A. Faulkner (1979) Histochemical characteristics of the masseter and temporalis muscles of the rhesus monkey *(Macaca mulatta).* Anat Rec *193:* 389–402.

Pette, D., R.S. Staron (1997) Mammalian skeletal muscle fiber type transitions. Int Rev Cytol *170:* 143–223.

Rubinstein, N.A., G.E. Lyons, A.M. Kelly (1988) Hormonal control of myosin heavy chain genes during development of skeletal muscles. Ciba Found Symp *138:* 35–51.

Rudnicki, M.A., G. Jackowski, L. Saggin, M.W. McBurney (1990) Actin and myosin expression during development of cardiac muscle from cultured embryonal carcinoma cells. Dev Biol *138:* 348–358.

Schiaffino, S., L. Gorza, S. Sartore, L. Saggin, S. Ausoni, M. Vianello, K. Gundersen, T. Lomo (1989) Three myosin heavy chain isoforms in type 2 skeletal muscle fibres. J Muscle Cell Motil *10:* 197–205.

Schiaffino, S., C. Reggiani (1996) Molecular diversity of myofibrillar proteins: Gene regulation and functional significance. Physiol Rev *76:* 371–423.

Walters, T.J., H.L. Sweeney, R.P. Farrar (1991) Influence of electrical stimulation on a fast-twitch muscle in aging rats. J Appl Physiol *71:* 1921–1928.

Widmer, C., D. Klugman, A. English (1997) Anatomical partitioning and nerve branch patterns in the adult rabbit masseter. Acta Anat *159:* 222–232.

Cells
Tissues
Organs

Cells Tissues Organs 2001;169:218–225

Properties of Sensory Neurons Innervating Synovial Joints

Peter Grigg

Department of Physiology, University of Massachusetts Medical School, Worcester, Mass., USA

Key Words
Joints · Afferents · Neurons

Abstract
While it is clear that the TMJ joint has a sensory innervation like other synovial joints, there is little specific information about the function of the innervation of the TMJ. In order to provide a template upon which future studies might build, this article briefly reviews the function of sensory neurons in other synovial joints.

Introduction

When a synovial joint is subjected to external loading, it rotates subject to constraints that are imposed by its soft tissue components. The ligaments and the fibrous capsule are deformed by joint rotations, and they develop stresses that oppose further rotation. The fibrous capsule (and to a lesser extent, the ligaments) of the joint are richly innervated by sensory (afferent) neurons that are mechanically sensitive. These neurons are activated by tensile stresses. Thus, joint rotations cause capsule loading, that activates afferent neurons in the joint capsule. The resulting activity in joint afferent neurons signals the nervous system that the joint is near its limit of rotation. Other sensory neurons found in soft tissues of joints are nociceptors – neurons that when activated mediate the sense of pain. They respond to multiple stimulus modalities, including very intense mechanical stimuli, all of which appear to play a role in mediating the sense of pain.

The focus of this volume is the temporo-mandibular joint (TMJ). It has been shown that, in human [Favia and Maiorano, 1995] and sheep [Tahmesebi-Sarvestani et al., 1996], the TMJ contains sensory end organs similar to those found in other synovial joints. It may be noted that in small animals such as mice, mostly free nerve endings are found in the TMJ [Dreessen et al., 1990]. Nonetheless, because of its inaccessibilty to study, little is known about the function of the innervation of the TMJ. Fortunately, there is a high level of homology in the properties of sensory neurons from other synovial joints such as knee, hip, ankle, and elbow. Thus, I shall describe what is known about the stimuli that activate sensory neurons in synovial joints and what use (if any) the nervous system makes use of the resulting information. I am promoting this as a model for afferents from the TMJ and, potentially for studying afferents from the TMJ.

In order to understand the behavior of sensory neurons that signal mechanical events in joint capsules, it is neces-

KARGER
Fax + 41 61 306 12 34
E-Mail karger@karger.ch
www.karger.com

Accessible online at:
www.karger.com/journals/cto

Peter Grigg, PhD
Department of Physiology S4-245
University of Massachusetts Medical School
55 Lake Ave, Worcester MA 01655 (USA)
Tel. +1 508 856 2457, Fax +1 508 856 5997, E-Mail Peter.Grigg@umassmed.edu

sary to understand the basic mechanics of the joint capsule and the role that it plays in constraining joint rotations. A joint capsule is a fibrous tissue structure that surrounds and encapsulates a synovial joint. Capsules are not uniform structures: they incorporate thickenings that function as ligaments as well as sheet – like regions that are relatively soft. When a joint is rotated into a limit of its rotation, the ligaments and capsule are stretched along one side of the joint, and are relaxed on the other. The limit of rotation of the joint is defined by the loads that are sustained by soft tissue structures. In the case of the knee, the posterior side of the joint – the side that is stretched on extension – appears to be well adapted to the tissue stretch that is caused by extension. It consists of a sheet of very soft tissue, that is coupled to the femur through a suspension cable arrangement [Grigg and Hoffman, 1989]. When the knee is rotated into the limit of extension, the posterior capsule is stretched along the direction of the long axis of the leg [Grigg and Hoffman, 1993]. Tensile strains and stresses are produced along that direction. It is an important finding that in the knee, the posterior capsule plays a relatively minor role in joint stabilization. In extension rotations, the loads that the posterior capsule imposes on the suspension cable are very low, on the order of 0.09 N/mm. The posterior capsule appears to sustain less than 4% of an extension moment about the knee [Grigg and Hoffman, 1993]. The mechanical role of other regions of the capsule, such as those that flank the patellar tendon in the knee, is less clear although they also appear to lack a major role.

Innervation of Joints

Nerve fibers enter the joint and terminate in soft tissues, mainly in the joint capsule. Two classes of sensory neurons make up the sensory innervation. One class consists of neurons with large, myelinated (group 2) axons; the second is made up of small diameter, unmyelinated or thinly myelinated (groups 3 and 4) axons, also known as 'fine' afferents. Group 2 sensory neurons innervate large, multicellular end organs that are located in the joint capsule. These units are mechanoreceptors; i.e., they are activated by mechanical stimuli. They have very low thresholds and high sensitivities.

The fine afferents are nociceptors (pain sensors). They have free nerve endings as terminals, have high thresholds for mechanical activation, and may be activated by multiple stimulus modalities. They are sensitized by repetitive activation or by treatment with algesic substances [Kanaka et al., 1985; Heppelmann et al., 1986; Schaible and Schmidt, 1988; Neugebauer et al., 1989; Schepelmann et al., 1992], and participate in neurogenic inflammation. Most are mechanically sensitive: intense, forceful rotations or indentation stimuli are required to activate them [Schaible and Schmidt, 1983a,b].

Morphology of Afferent Neurons

The connection between a nerve ending with a particular morphology, demonstrated in experiments on fixed and stained material, and electrophysiological recordings of afferents with particular response properties has been made only indirectly for joint afferents. The model that I am presenting here appears to be most generally accepted.

Group 2 Afferents

Ruffini-Type Endings

The parent axon enters the joint capsule, divides, and terminates in large terminal processes inside multicellular end-organ structures (fig. 1) [Boyd, 1954]. These consist of a number of nerve processes that envelop and contact bundles of collagen fibers with a particular orientation [Halata, 1977]. Ruffini endings are found primarily in capsule regions that are subjected to tensile loading, such as the posterior side of the knee capsule, and they are activated by stretch stimuli. Stretch stimuli, however, generate both tensile stresses and strains. Fuller et al. [1991] showed that responses of capsule afferent were associated with tensile loads (i.e. stresses) in the capsule, with only a minor relationship to tensile strain. Thus, capsule mechanoreceptors can be thought of as load cells that detect tensile loads or stresses in the joint's fibrous capsule. Furthermore, they are driven by very small tensile stresses. For example, group 2 afferents in the posterior side of the joint capsule are activated when tensile stresses in the capsule reach about 15–20 kPa [Khalsa et al., 1996]. When an intact knee joint is rotated into extension, the discharge of Ruffini afferents is proportional to the load applied to the joint [Grigg and Greenspan, 1977] (fig. 2). This follows, since the capsule is one of the structures that, however minimally, resists extension. Responses are elicited in afferents only when the knee is near the limit of rotation in extension; for this reason, these afferents have been hypothesized to be limit detectors [Grigg and Hoffman 1982].

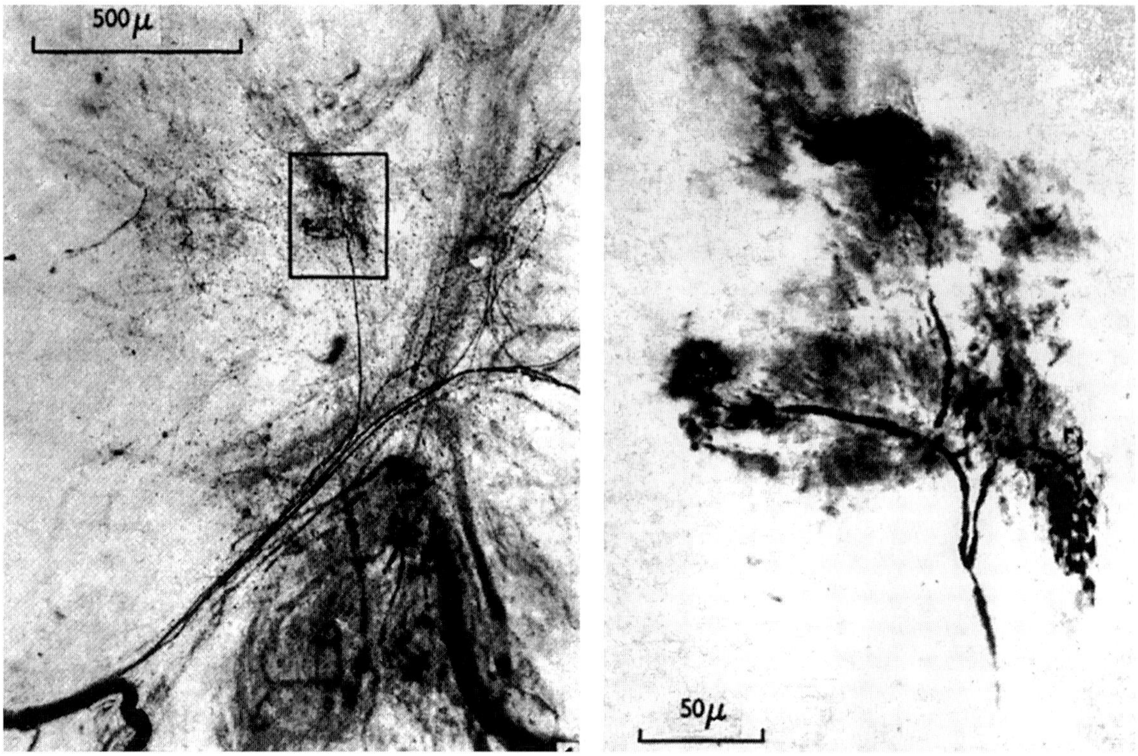

Fig. 1. Micrograph of gold chloride stained posterior joint capsule, showing sensory nerve processes. Left panel: low power. Right panel: higher magnification of the area outlined in the left panel. From Boyd [1954].

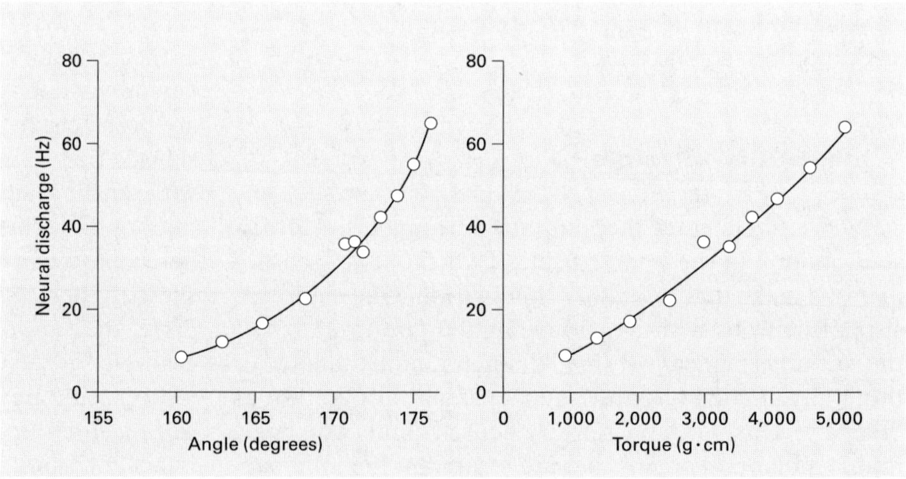

Fig. 2. Neural response of single knee capsule afferent from monkey, in response to knee extension. Left panel: Response plotted vs. joint angle, where 180 degrees is full extension. Right panel: Same response plotted vs. joint moment. From Grigg and Greenspan [1977].

Lamellar (Paciniform) Afferents

A second population of group 2 afferents innervates a thin, lamellar bulb structure referred to as the 'paciniform' or 'Golgi-Mazzoni' ending (fig. 3). In the knee, these are mainly located in the capsule along the sides of the patellar tendon, where the capsule is shielded from tensile loads.

Lamellar endings have been shown to be poorly activated by rotations of the joint [Grigg et al., 1982]. Furthermore they have been shown, in studies based on in

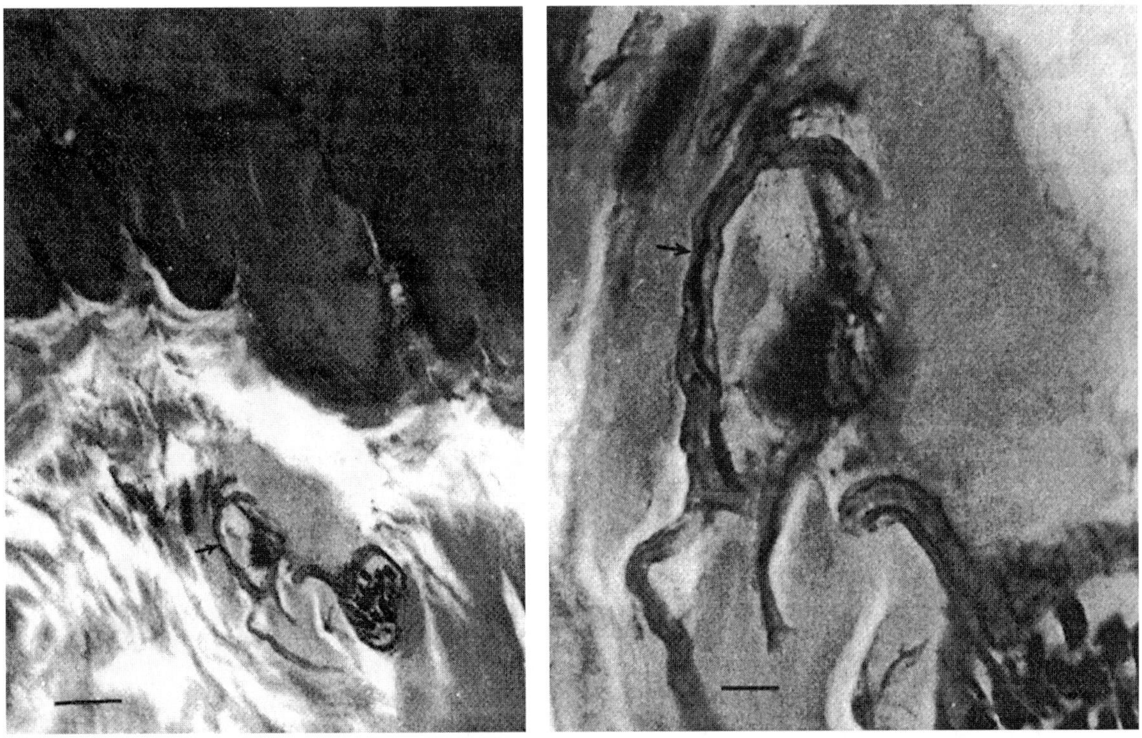

Fig. 3. Micrograph of gold chloride stained joint capsule from medial side of the knee joint in cat. Left panel: Low power; scale = 200 µm. Nerve processes are located in fibro-adipose tissue beneath the capsule (arrow). Right panel: High magnification of lamellar sensory nerve ending. Scale = 50 µm. From Grigg et al. [1982].

vitro observations, to be insensitive to tensile loading. Rather, they are activated by compression stimuli, such as by external stimuli compressing the capsule surface, or by increases in hydrostatic pressure [Grigg et al., 1982].

Fine Afferents

Group 3 and 4 afferents have many properties in common, so I am discussing them together. Group 4 axons are unmyelinated, also known as c-fibers. They conduct action potentials at velocities of 1 m/s or less. Group 3 axons, also referred to as Aδ fibers, are thinly myelinated, and conduct action potentials at velocities of 2–15 m/s. The axons may branch near their sensory terminals, and a given axon may have receptive endings that are as much as 15 mm apart. The sensory terminal of each branch is a fine, unmyelinated tip that has, over its last 100 µm, the lumpy appearance of a string of beads [Heppelmann et al., 1988]. The lumps are thought to be individual receptive sites. Most c fiber terminals contain vesicles of substance P and calcitonin-gene related peptide (CGRP), peptides that are released on activation [Ferrell and Russell, 1986] and are involved in inflammatory responses.

Fine afferents innervate all of the soft tissue components of the joint, including the capsule, the collateral ligaments, and the patellar tendon. Fine afferents can be directly stimulated by applying compression stimuli directly to the appropriate location (i.e., the receptive field). Large compression forces are required in order to activate fine afferents, and receptive fields are spot-like [Schaible and Schmidt, 1983]. Single afferents may have several active spots, reflecting axonal branching. Most fine afferents can also be activated by rotations of the knee. Very intense, forceful rotations, into the limits of movement, are required, and individual afferents are excited by multiple types of rotations such as external, internal, or extension rotations [Schaible and Schmidt, 1983] (fig. 4).

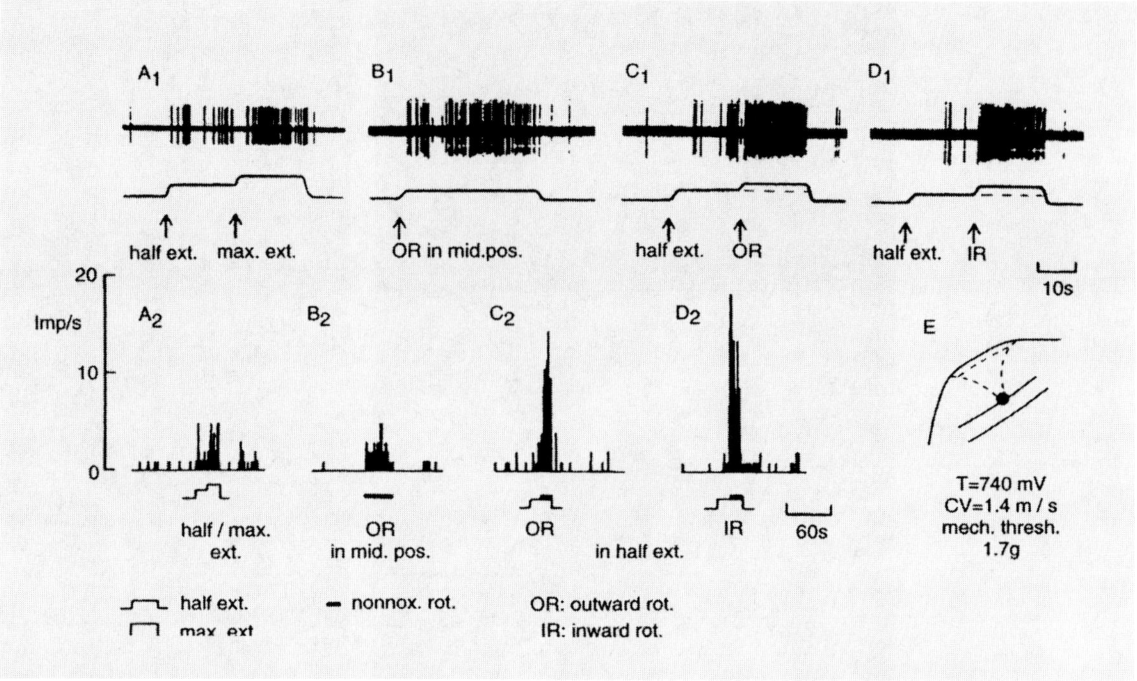

Fig. 4. Responses of a single group 4 afferent neuron to a variety of rotational movements of the cat knee. The location of the spot-like receptive filed is shown in **E**. **A**, **B**, **C**, and **D** illustrate the responses of the neuron to: (**A**) rotations of the knee into extension; (**B**) into outward rotation with the joint in midrange of flexion; (**C**) into outward rotation with knee extended, and (**D**) into inward rotation. The same data are plotted as raw traces (above) and as histograms (below). Maximal rotations were considered to be noxious. From Schaible and Schmidt [1983].

Reflexes Mediated by Joint Afferents

It has been long postulated that sensory neurons in joints play a role in regulating movements of the joints. However, the previous studies dealing with this phenomenon have been sufficiently flawed that practically nothing can be concluded about it. For example, it is abundantly clear that when joint afferent neurons are activated, excitability changes can be observed in motor units acting around joints. However, there are several problems in interpreting the literature dealing with this phenomenon. First, most studies have used electrical stimuli applied to joint nerves. However, because electrical stimuli excite afferents in unnatural combinations, and may excite A and C fibers together, the results of such experiments are not interpretable beyond concluding that some afferents can influence the excitability of some motoneurons. Even when joint reflexes have been elicited with natural stimuli such as joint rotation or capsule indentation [Grigg et al., 1978; Ferrell et al., 1990], the results are still difficult to interpret. The basic problem is that peripheral reflexes may not be simple, with single actions. For example, it has been shown [Duysens and Pearson, 1976] that cutaneous reflexes in the limbs of quadrupeds have different effects depending on where in the step cycle they are elicited. Reflex effects elicited by cutaneous stimuli are different when they are applied during the stance phase vs. the swing phase of walking. Thus it may be an oversimplification to assume that activation of joint afferents might elicit a simple reflex. If joint reflexes are, like cutaneous reflexes, dependent on their timing within a step cycle, then the previous reports of joint reflexes, whether they were elicited by natural or electrical stimuli, cannot be simply interpreted. It should also be noted that in the TMJ, where movements may not be as stereotypical as in locomotion, the situation may be altogether different.

Reflexes Mediated by Fine Afferents

Fine afferents in joints appear to have simple reflex actions: when activated they elicit limb flexion. Demonstrating such reflexes is complicated because stimuli that would activate fine afferents will also activate group 2 afferents, thus confounding the effects of the two. He et al. [1988] resolved this issue by taking advantage of the sensitization phenomenon in nociceptors. The knee joint was rotated gently and excitability changes were sought by recording from a flexor motoneuron. In the initial state, joint rotation elicited no response from the motoneuron. Then the knee joint was inflamed by injecting it with kaolin and carrageenan. This treatment caused an inflammation, which is known to sensitize fine afferents. Thus, gentle rotation of the inflamed knee would excite fine afferents. When the rotation was repeated after the inflammation, it caused excitation of the flexor motoneuron. This means that nociceptor neurons mediate limb flexion (i.e. a flexion reflex), a common role for nociceptors.

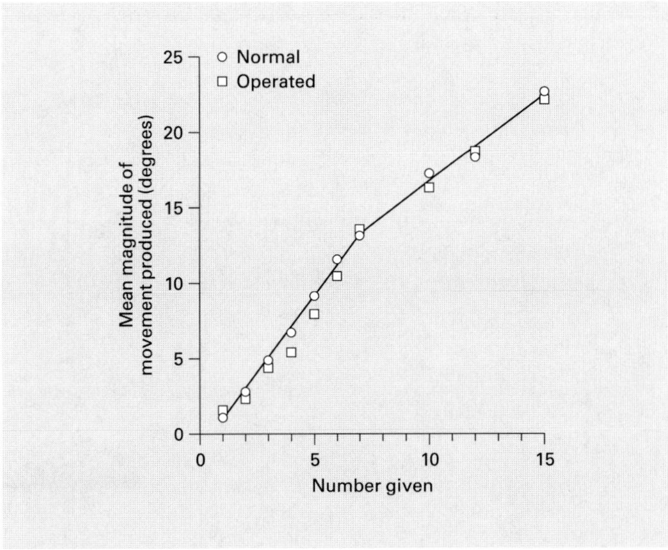

Fig. 5. Ability of human subjects to generate movements of a desired magnitude. The task was to abduct the hip joint to a target angle without visual guidance. Number given: Target angle assigned to the subject. Magnitude of movement produced: actual abduction movement achieved by subject. The subject had a hip replacement, with a total excision of the capsule, on the operated side, and a relatively normal joint on the normal side. From Grigg et al. [1973].

Role of Joint Afferents in Proprioception

Proprioception refers to the senses of movement and position of a joint. Its basis is in the responses of neurons that innervate structures in and around a limb. Those neurons, when activated appropriately, mediate the sense of proprioception. Relevant to the present discussion is the issue of the relative contribution made by afferents from joints. It is generally accepted that when the joint is in the middle of its range of movement, proprioception is mediated by activity in afferent neurons from muscles acting across the joint [Proske et al., 1988]. In subjects in which the knee joint capsule is anesthetized [Clark, 1979] or in patients in whom the hip joint capsule has been excised in a total joint replacement procedure [Grigg et al., 1973], minimal effects were seen in proprioception (fig. 5). In knees, afferents from the posterior capsule are activated only when the joint is forcefully rotated into extension, past an angle of about 165 degrees. Those results suggest that joint afferents that are activated by extension act as limit detectors, mediating a sense that the joint is at or near its limit of rotation.

Table 1. Magnitudes of cartilage lesions observed in dog knee joints, 72 weeks after treatment

Treatment	Severity of cartilage lesion					
	0	1	2	3	4	5
Control	XX					
Joint nerves cut	XX					
ACL transected		XX	XX			
ACL transection plus joint nerves cut			X	X	XX	XX

Cartilage lesions are ordered from 0 (normal cartilage) to 5 (fragmentation of the cartilage and exposure of the sub-chondral bone). From O'Connor et al. [1992].

Role of Joint Afferent Neurons in an Unstable Joint

O'Connor and his colleagues [O'Connor et al., 1992, 1993] have shown that knee joint afferents play an important role in protecting knees that are mechanically unstable. They destabilized knee joints in dogs, by cutting the anterior cruciate ligament (ACL) unilaterally. The dogs were allowed to survive, and to move about freely, for as long as 1.5 years. Upon sacrifice, it was shown that cartilage lesions typical of osteoarthritis were observed in all of the dogs whose ACL was cut. Importantly, however, the degree of cartilage injury was dependent on whether or not the joint nerves had been cut or left intact. Leaving the joint nerves intact at the time of ACL section protected the joint from injury, while cutting the joint nerves prior to or coincident with ACL section biased the outcome in favor of greater cartilage lesions (table 1). The key factor

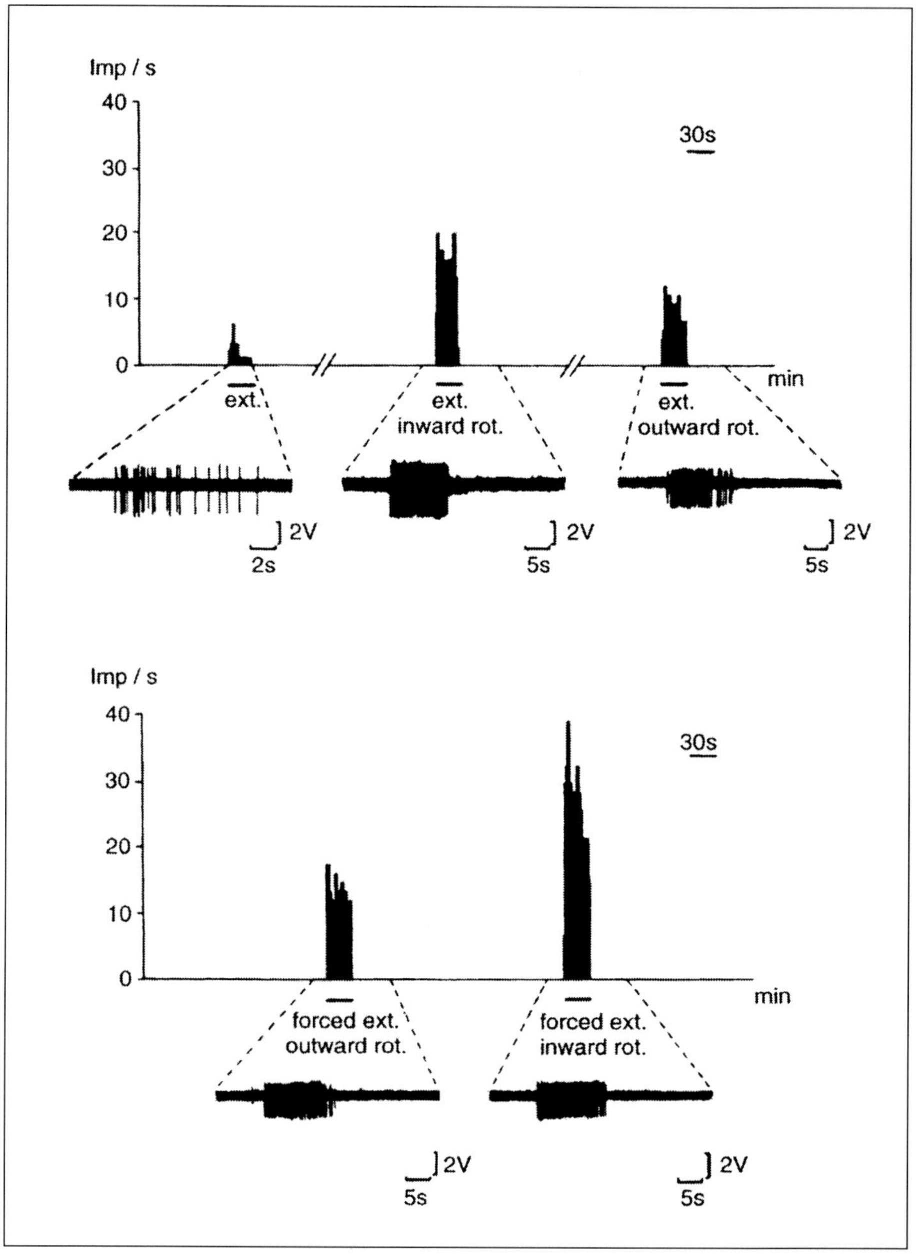

Fig. 6. Responses of a single group 2 afferent neuron originating from the anterior cruciate ligament, in cat knee. The lack of specificity of this neuron to rotations in different directions is illustrated. Responses (shown both as raw data traces and as histograms) are recorded in relation to rotations in a variety of directions (indicated in figure). From Krauspe et al. [1992].

in protection of the joint is having afferent (sensory) inflow present at the time that the joint becomes unstable. These results are consistent with the model that the animal uses sensory information from the joint nerves to detect extreme rotations, or movements that produce large tissue loads. This information allows the animal to adopt movement strategies that minimize damage, protecting the joint. This model is consistent with what is known about both fine afferents and Ruffini type afferents, in that fine afferents signal that a joint has been rotated into some extreme, noxious angle and Ruffini afferents signal that the joint is rotated into a limit of its range of movement.

Mechanoreceptor Neurons in Ligaments

Sensory neurons have been described in ligaments, most notably in the ACL of the knee [Krauspe et al., 1992]. In a recent study, responses of afferent neurons from the ACL were recorded while the knee was rotated. It was shown that individual afferents lack directional specificity: they were activated by rotations into extension, by inward and outward rotation, and combinations of the above [Krauspe et al., 1992] (fig. 6). This lack of specificity means that they cannot play a role in signaling anything other than extreme rotations. The same lack of specificity also makes them a poor candidate for being involved in reflexes that might somehow be a part of motor control.

Acknowledgements

Preparation of this paper was supported by NIH grant NS-10783.

References

Boyd, I.A. (1954) The histological structure of the receptors in the knee-joint of the cat correlated with their physiological response. J Physiol *124:* 476–488.

Clark, F.J., K.W. Horch, S.M. Bach, G.F. Larson (1979) Contribution of cutaneous and joint receptors to static knee-position sense in man. J Neurophysiol *42:* 877–888.

Dreessen, D., Z. Halata, T. Strasmann (1990) Sensory innervation of the temperomandibular joint in the mouse. Acta Anat *139:* 154–160.

Duysens, J., K.G. Pearson (1976) The role of cutaneous afferents from the distal hindlimb in the regulation of the step cycle of thalamic cats. Exp Brain Res *24:* 245–255.

Favia, G., E. Maiorano (1995) Presence of neuroreceptors in normal and diseased temperomandibular joints. Boll Soc Ital Biol Sper *71:* 201–212.

Ferrell, W.R. J.R. Rosenberg, R.H. Baxendale (1990) Fourier analysis of the relation between the discharge of quadriceps motor units and periodic mechanical stimulation of cat knee receptors. Exp Physiol *75:* 739–750.

Ferrell, W.R., N.J. Russell (1986) Extravasation in the knee induced by antidromic stimulation of articular C fibre afferents of the anaesthetized cat. J Physiol (Lond) *379:* 407–416.

Fuller, M.S., P. Grigg, A.H., Hoffman (1991) Response of joint capsule neurons to axial stress and strain during dynamic loading in cat. J Neurophysiol *65:* 1321–1328.

Grigg, P. (1975) Mechanical factors influencing response of joint afferent neurons from cat knee. J Neurophysiol *38:* 1473–1484.

Grigg, P., G.A. Finerman, L.H. Riley (1973) Joint-position sense after total hip replacement. J Bone Joint Surg [Am] *55:* 1016–1125.

Grigg, P., B.J. Greenspan (1977) Response of primate joint afferent neurons to mechanical stimulation of knee joint. J Neurophysiol *40:* 1–8.

Grigg, P., E.P. Harrigan, K.E. Fogarty (1978) Segmental reflexes mediated by joint afferent neurons in cat knee. J Neurophysiol *41:* 9–14.

Grigg, P., A.H. Hoffman (1982) Properties of Ruffini afferents revealed by stress analysis of isolated sections of cat knee capsule. J Neurophysiol *47:* 41–54.

Grigg, P., A.H. Hoffman (1989) Calibrating joint capsule mechanoreceptors as in vivo soft tissue load cells. J Biomech *22:* 781–785.

Grigg, P., A.H. Hoffman (1993) Loading and deformation of the cat posterior knee joint capsule in axial and extension rotations. J Biochem *26:* 1283–1290.

Grigg, P., A.H. Hoffman, K.E. Fogarty (1982) Properties of Golgi-Mazzoni afferents in cat knee joint capsule, as revealed by mechanical studies of isolated joint capsule. J Neurophysiol *47:* 31–40.

Halata, Z. (1977) The ultrastructure of the sensory nerve endings in the articular capsule of the domestic cat (Ruffini corpuscles and Pacinian corpuscles). J Anat *124:* 717–729.

He, X., U. Proske, H.G. Schaible, R.F. Schmidt (1988) Acute inflammation of the knee joint in the cat alters responses of flexor motoneurons to leg movement. J Neurophysiol *59:* 326–340.

Heppelmann, B., C. Heuss, R.F. Schmidt (1988) Fiber size distribution of myelinated and unmyelinated axons in the medial and posterior articular nerves of the cat's knee joint. Somatosens Res *5:* 273–281.

Heppelmann, B., A. Pfeffer, H.G. Schaible, R.F. Schmidt (1986) Effects of acetylsalicylic acid and indomethacin on single groups III and IV sensory units from acutely inflamed joints. Pain *26:* 337–351.

Kanaka, R., H.G. Schaible, R.F. Schmidt (1985) Activation of fine articular afferent units by bradykinin. Brain Res *327:* 81–90.

Khalsa, P.S. A.H.Hoffman, P. Grigg (1996) Mechanical states encoded by stretch-sensitive neurons in feline joint capsule. J Neurophysiol *76:* 175–187.

Krauspe, R., M. Schmidt, H.G. Schaible (1992) Sensory innervation of the anterior cruciate ligament: An electrophysiological study of the response properties of single identified mechanoreceptors in the cat. J Bone Joint Surg [Am] *74:* 390–397.

Neugebauer, V., H.G. Schaible, R.F. Schmidt (1989) Sensitization of articular afferents to mechanical stimuli by bradykinin. Pflügers Arch *415:* 330–335.

O'Connor, B.L., D.M. Visco, K.D. Brandt, M. Albrecht, A.B. O'Connor (1993) Sensory nerves only temporarily protect the unstable canine knee joint from osteoarthritis: Evidence that sensory nerves reprogram the central nervous system after cruciate ligament transection. Arthritis Rheum *36:* 1154–1163.

O'Connor, B.L., D.M. Visco, K.D. Brandt, S.L. Myers, L.A. Kalasinski (1992) Neurogenic acceleration of osteoarthrosis: The effects of previous neurectomy of the articular nerves on the development of osteoarthrosis after transection of the anterior cruciate ligament in dogs. J Bone Joint Surg [Am] *74:* 367–376.

Proske, U., H.G. Schaible, R.F. Schmidt (1988) Joint receptors and kinaesthesia. Exp Brain Res *72:* 219–224.

Schaible, H.G., R.F. Schmidt (1983a) Activation of groups III and IV sensory units in medial articular nerve by local mechanical stimulation of knee joint. J Neurophysiol *49:* 35–44.

Schaible, H.G., R.F. Schmidt (1983b) Responses of fine medial articular nerve afferents to passive movements of knee joints. J Neurophysiol *49:* 1118–1126.

Schaible, H.G., R.F. Schmidt (1988) excitation and sensitization of fine articular afferents from cat's knee joint by prostaglandin E_2. J Physiol (Lond) *403:* 91–104.

Schepelmann, K. K. Messlinger, H.H. Schaible, R.F. Schmidt (1992) Inflammatory mediators and nociception in the joint: Excitation and sensitization of slowly conducting afferent fibers of cat's knee by prostaglandin I2. Neuroscience *50:* 237–247.

Tahmasebi-Sarvestani, A., R.A. Tedman, A. Gross (1996) Neural structures within the sheep temperomandibular joint. J Orofacial Pain *10:* 217–231.

Cells
Tissues
Organs

Cells Tissues Organs 2001;169:226–237

Sex Differences in Brainstem Neural Activation after Injury to the TMJ Region

David A. Bereiter

Departments of Neuroscience and Surgery, Brown University School of Medicine, Rhode Island Hospital, Providence, R.I., USA

Key Words

Cervical spinal cord · c-*fos* gene · Sex differences · Temporomandibular joint · Trigeminal spinal nucleus

Abstract

The basis for a higher prevalence of painful temporomandibular disorders (TMD) among women than men is not known. The present study used Fos-like immunoreactivity (Fos-LI) to quantify the pattern and magnitude of neural activation within the trigeminal brainstem complex of male and female rats caused by acute inflammatory injury to the temporomandibular joint (TMJ) region. Also, Fos-LI was assessed in animals given morphine, a preferential mu opioid receptor agonist, or U50,488H, a selective kappa opioid agonist, prior to TMJ injury to determine if opioid modulation of neural activation was similar in males and females. The general pattern of Fos-LI after TMJ injury was similar in males and females. This pattern was characterized by a high density of Fos-positive neurons in the dorsal paratrigeminal nucleus (dPa5), subnucleus interpolaris/caudalis transition region (Vi/Vc-vl), and in the superficial laminae at the subnucleus caudalis/upper cervical spinal cord (Vc/C2) junction ipsilateral to TMJ injury. In contrast to other regions the number of Fos-positive neurons produced at the Vc/C2 junction was proportional to the concentration of mustard oil injected into the TMJ region. In addition, proestrus females produced higher levels of Fos-LI at the Vc/C2 junction than diestrus females or males. Morphine caused a greater dose-related reduction in Fos-LI at the dPa5 and Vc/C2 junction in males than females. By contrast, U50,488H caused a dose-related reduction in Fos-LI only at the Vc/C2 junction of proestrus females. These results support the hypothesis that the Vc/C2 junction region plays a critical role in the integration of pain signals originating from the TMJ region and may underlie sex differences in sensory processing related to TMJ pain.

Abbreviations used in this paper

dPa5	dorsal paratrigeminal nucleus
Fos-LI	Fos-like immunoreactivity
TMD	temporomandibular disorders
TMJ	temporomandibular joint
U50,488H	selective kappa opioid receptor agonist
Vc/C2	trigeminal subnucleus caudalis/upper cervical spinal cord junction region
Vi/Vc-vl	trigeminal subnucleus interpolaris/caudalis transition region, ventrolateral portion

KARGER

Fax + 41 61 306 12 34
E-Mail karger@karger.ch
www.karger.com

Accessible online at:
www.karger.com/journals/cto

David A. Bereiter, PhD
Departments of Surgery and Neuroscience, Brown University School of Medicine
Rhode Island Hospital, 222 Nursing Arts Bldg.
Providence, RI 02903 (USA)
Tel. +1 401 444 4277, Fax +1 401 444 8052, E-Mail dbereiter@lifespan.org

Introduction

Temporomandibular disorders (TMD) represent a heterogeneous group of painful conditions that involve the temporomandibular joint (TMJ) region and muscles of mastication with frequent spreading to adjacent regions of the head and neck [Stohler, 1995]. The basis for TMD pain is not known although symptoms such as the spreading of pain, pain referral to other craniofacial regions, and enhanced sensitivity to other experimentally induced pains [Maixner et al., 1995a, 1998], suggest the involvement of central neural mechanisms.

The TMJ region is innervated by a complex network of fibers originating from trigeminal, upper cervical spinal, and vagal sensory ganglion neurons [Klineberg, 1971; Denny-Brown and Yanagisawa, 1973; Widenfalk and Wiberg, 1990; Kido et al., 1993; Uddman et al., 1998]. The widespread overlap of peripheral fields and central projection from these sensory neurons likely contributes to the poor localization of TMD pain. Accordingly, extensive convergence from trigeminal, cervical spinal and vagal sources onto second-order brainstem neurons has confounded the identification of the central neural pathways necessary for TMD pain. Quantitative immunostaining for Fos (Fos-LI), the protein product of the immediate early gene, c-*fos*, is well suited to assess the pattern of central neural activation by acute injury to tissues supplied by multiple nerves such as the TMJ region. Fos-LI provides a stable signal to assess a neuronal population response, but with single cell resolution, an experimental advantage not readily achieved by other methods such as electrophysiology or neural imaging. For models involving acute pain Fos immunostaining has proved a reliable and useful marker for nociceptor-evoked neural activity in the spinal dorsal horn [Hunt et al., 1987; Bullitt, 1990] and caudal brainstem [Lu et al., 1993; Strassman and Vos, 1993; Meng and Bereiter, 1996].

Previously, we determined that acute injury to the TMJ region produced Fos-positive neurons in several spatially discrete regions of the trigeminal spinal nucleus and upper cervical dorsal horn of male rats [Hathaway et al., 1995; Bereiter and Bereiter, 2000]. However, it is not known if Fos-LI produced by TMJ injury is similar for males and females. Endocrine status is a recognized risk factor in TMD [Stohler, 1997] and women of reproductive age seek treatment for TMD pain more often than postmenopausal women or men [LeResche, 1997; LeResche et al., 1997]. Thus, the primary aim of the present study was to compare the pattern and magnitude of Fos-LI produced by TMJ injury in males to that of females at different stages of the estrous cycle. Reduction in Fos-LI by analgesic drugs is an important line of evidence in support of c-*fos* gene expression as a marker for nociceptive spinal neurons [Presley et al., 1990; Hammond et al., 1992; Bereiter, 1997]. Since a reduced capacity to recruit endogenous opioid-dependent pain control pathways may contribute to the lower pain thresholds seen in some TMD patients [Maixner et al., 1995b], a second aim of this study was to determine if the opioid receptor agonists, morphine and the selective kappa opioid receptor agonist, U50,488H, had similar effects on Fos-LI produced in males and females after TMJ injury.

Materials and Methods

The experimental protocols were approved by the Institutional Animal Care and Use Committee of Rhode Island Hospital and conformed to the established guidelines set by The National Institute of Health guide for the care and use of laboratory animals [Publications No. 86–23, revised 1985].

Experimental Design

Adult male and female rats (250–370 g, Sprague-Dawley, Harlan) were anesthetized with pentobarbital sodium (65 mg/kg i.p.). Catheters were placed in the jugular vein (drugs) and the femoral artery (arterial pressure) and skin incisions were infiltrated with 2% lidocaine jelly. Body temperature was kept at 38 °C. The stage of the estrous cycle was determined from vaginal smear cytology followed over several days prior to the experiment to ensure a normal cycle. Two experimental designs were used to compare the number of Fos-positive neurons produced in males, proestrus females, and diestrus females. In the first series, different concentrations of the selective small fiber excitant, mustard oil (0.2, 2 or 20% allyl isothiocyanate in mineral oil, 25 µl) were injected into the left TMJ region of males and proestrus females. Diestrus females received 20% mustard oil injections only. Sudan black dye was added to the injectate to aid in localizing the site of injection. Vehicle controls received saline injection (0% mustard oil, 25 µl) into the TMJ region. In a second series, males, proestrus females and diestrus females received injections of 20% mustard oil alone into the TMJ region or 20% mustard oil plus pretreatment with one of the following opioid-related drugs: morphine sulfate (Marcam), a preferential mu opioid agonist; naloxone hydrochloride (Sigma), a nonselective opioid receptor antagonist; U50,488H (NIDA supply program), a selective kappa opioid agonist; and nor-binaltorphimine (nor-BNI, NIDA drug supply program), selective kappa opioid receptor antagonist. All drugs were dissolved in 0.9% saline and dosage was calculated on the basis of the weight of the salt form of the drug. Animals were given a single dose of drug intravenously 15 min prior to injection of 20% mustard oil into the TMJ region. For animals that received opioid receptor antagonist plus agonist, the antagonist was given 10 min prior to the agonist and followed 15 min later by 20% mustard oil into the TMJ region. The drug dosages were: morphine 0.03, 0.3, 3 and 7 mg/kg and 3 mg/kg plus 1 mg/kg naloxone; U50,488H 0.03, 0.3, 3, 7 mg/kg and 3 mg/kg plus 16 mg/kg nor-binaltorphimine. The number of animals in each treatment group ranged from four to seven. Additional groups of males and proestrus females served as surgical and drug controls and received no injection into the TMJ region: surgical preparation alone (NS group), morphine alone (7 mg/kg), and U50,488H alone (7 mg/kg). In separate groups of male and proestrus females 2% Evan's blue was given i.v. 10 min before transcardiac perfusion, approximately 1.5 h after TMJ injury (20% mustard oil), to estimate the extent of local inflammation, after dye extraction from the surrounding TMJ tissues and measured spectrophotometrically [Haas et al., 1992].

Fos Immunocytochemistry

Animals remained anesthetized for 2 h after TMJ injury, then given a bolus injection of pentobarbital (60 mg/kg i.v.), perfused through the heart with heparinized saline, followed by 250 ml cold fixative (4% paraformaldehyde, 0.02% picric acid in 0.1 *M* phosphate buffer, pH 7.4). The caudal brainstem and adjacent cervical spinal cord was removed and postfixed for 1 h. Transverse sections (50 µm) were cut on a vibratome and collected in cold 0.01 *M* phosphate-buffered saline (PBS). Brain sections were incubated in 5% normal donkey serum (30 min), followed by affinity-purified rabbit polyclonal anti-Fos antibody (Ab-2, Oncogene Science; 1:15,000, 40 h at 4°C), biotinylated donkey antirabbit antibodies (Chemicon; 1:300, 105 min) and avidin-biotin-peroxidase complex (Vector; 60 min). Fos-positive neuronal nuclei were visualized by incubation in a nickel-cobalt diaminobenzidine solution activated by 0.01% hydrogen peroxide. After rinsing in PBS, sections were mounted on untreated glass slides, air dried and coverslipped with mounting medium. Under bright-field illumination, Fos-positive neuronal nuclei were distinguished as homogenous gray-black elements with a well-defined border. Specific staining was abolished by omission of primary antiserum.

Data Analysis

The approximate rostrocaudal level of each brainstem section was noted and categorized at 500 µm intervals from 2 mm rostral to 7 mm caudal to the obex. The obex is a surface landmark defined by the caudal end of the fourth ventricle approximately 500 µm rostral to the most caudal tip of trigeminal subnucleus interpolaris [Yoshida et al., 1991]. Sixty to 70 sections per animal were counted at 100× magnification without prior knowledge of treatment. To facilitate statistical comparisons across multiple treatments, the mean number of Fos-positive neurons was determined for the following brainstem regions: (1) dorsal paratrigeminal region (dPa5, +0.5 to –0.5 mm relative to the obex), located along the dorsolateral edge of the main body of the trigeminal spinal nucleus and within the spinal trigeminal tract (see fig. 2, level 0 mm); (2) ventrolateral pole of the subnucleus interpolaris/caudalis transition region (Vi/Vc-vl, +0.5 to –1.0 mm) (see fig. 2, level 0 mm), and (3) junction region of the caudal Vc and the C2 segment of the cervical spinal cord (Vc/C2, –4.5 to –6.5 mm) (see fig. 2, level –6 mm). The superficial laminae (I-II) of Vc and upper cervical dorsal horn were distinguished from deeper laminae (III-V) as a zone that changed from a homogeneous to heterogeneous [Molander et al., 1989]. (4) Fos-positive nuclei also were counted in the caudal ventrolateral medulla (CVLM) located +0.5 to –1.0 mm relative to obex (see fig. 2, level 0 mm). The CVLM region, an important brainstem region for control of autonomic function [Dampney, 1994], appeared as a relatively compact cell group ventral to nucleus ambiguus, dorsal to the lateral reticular nucleus, medial to the trigeminal spinal nucleus, and lateral to the inferior olive. Cell counts were compared across treatment groups and ipsilateral versus contralateral to the TMJ injection by two-way analysis of variance. Individual comparisons were made by the Newman-Keuls test after analysis of variance [Winer, 1971]. Total cells produced within the trigeminal spinal nucleus and upper cervical dorsal horn was calculated from the cell counts corrected for the number of sections counted at each 500-µm segment over the rostrocaudal distance of +2 to –7 mm relative to the obex. The term Fos-LI is used interchangeably and meant to be synonymous with Fos-positive neuronal nuclei.

Results

General Distribution of Fos-LI after Injury to the TMJ Region

Acute injury to the TMJ region by mustard oil produced Fos-LI at caudal levels of the trigeminal spinal nucleus and upper cervical dorsal horn as shown in figure 1. Ipsilateral to TMJ injury Fos-LI appeared as two broad peaks of immunoreactive neuronal nuclei: at periobex levels and the spinomedullary junction, while neurons produced in the contralateral hemisphere were seen only at the level of the obex. Males and females displayed a similar general pattern of Fos-LI after injection of 20% mustard oil into the TMJ region; however, proestrus females produced significantly ($p < 0.001$) more Fos-positive neurons at periobex levels and at the spinomedullary junction than diestrus females or males. Over the rostrocaudal levels shown in figure 1, the calculated total number of Fos-positive neurons produced within the trigeminal spinal nucleus and upper cervical dorsal horn ipsilateral to the 20% mustard oil stimulus averaged 6,347 ± 802, 4,690 ± 749, and 3,895 ± 439 cells for proestrus females, diestrus females and males, respectively.

Concentration of Mustard Oil and Fos-LI in Specific Neuronal Cell Groups

A high density of Fos-positive neurons was produced in each of three spatially discrete regions of the trigeminal spinal nucleus and upper cervical spinal cord as highlighted by the boxed areas in figure 2. At periobex levels Fos-positive neurons were clustered bilaterally at the dPa5 and the Vi/Vc-vl transition region. Fewer neurons were produced in mid-portions of Vc (–2 to –4 mm to obex), while the greatest number of Fos-positive neurons was found in laminae I-II at the Vc/C2 junction region. Few Fos-positive cells (<5 per section) were seen in deeper laminae of Vc proper or at the Vc/C2 junction region. The effects of different concentrations of mustard oil on Fos-LI in the dPa5, Vi/Vc-vl transition region and laminae I-II of the Vc/C2 junction region are summarized in figure 3. In unstimulated controls (NS group) Fos-LI was

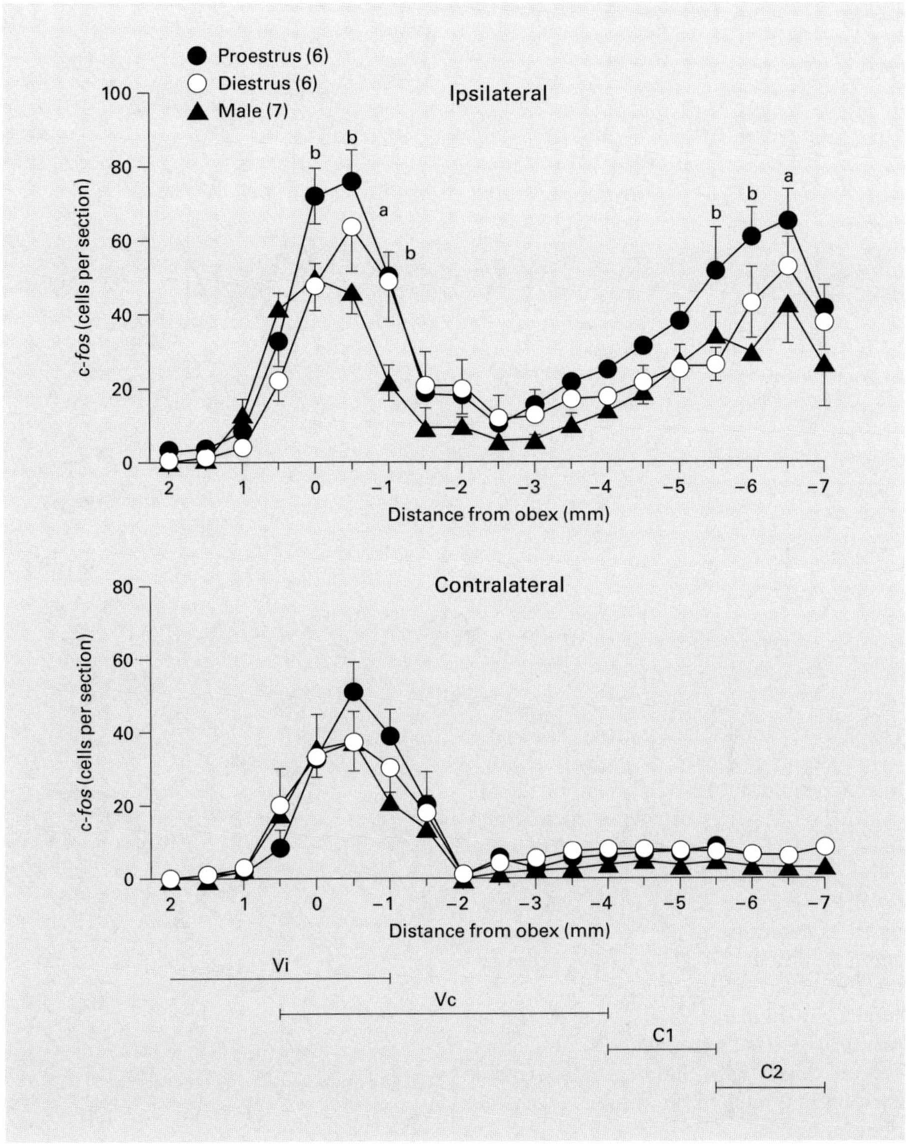

Fig. 1. Mean number of Fos-positive neurons produced within the trigeminal spinal nucleus and upper cervical dorsal horn after injection of mustard oil (20% solution, 25 μl) into the TMJ region expressed as a function of the distance from the obex. [a] $p < 0.05$, [b] $p < 0.01$ versus males. C1 = First cervical segment; C2 = second cervical segment; Vc = trigeminal subnucleus caudalis; Vi = trigeminal subnucleus interpolaris.

sparse in the dPa5 (fig. 3, upper panel) of proestrus females and males. Saline (0%) or 0.2% mustard oil injection into the TMJ region had little effect on Fos-LI produced ipsilateral to TMJ injury at the dPa5, while 2 and 20% mustard oil caused significant and similar increases in Fos-LI in proestrus females. Males displayed an increase in Fos-LI above controls only after 20% mustard oil. Note that diestrus females showed an increase in Fos-LI after 20% mustard oil similar to that of proestrus females and males. At the Vi/Vc-vl transition region (fig. 3, middle panel) Fos-LI increased significantly and similarly after injection of saline or mustard oil, independent of concentration, in proestrus females and males. By contrast, at the Vc/C2 junction region (fig. 3, lower panel) Fos-LI increased progressively with increasing concentrations of mustard oil in proestrus females and males. In addition, proestrus females produced a greater number of Fos-positive neurons than males after 0.2% ($p < 0.05$), 2% ($p < 0.01$) or 20% mustard oil compared to males ($p < 0.01$) and after 20% mustard oil compared to diestrus females ($p < 0.01$).

Effect of Morphine on Fos-LI in Specific Neuronal Cell Groups

To determine if opioid analgesics affected c-*fos* expression similarly in females and males, different doses of

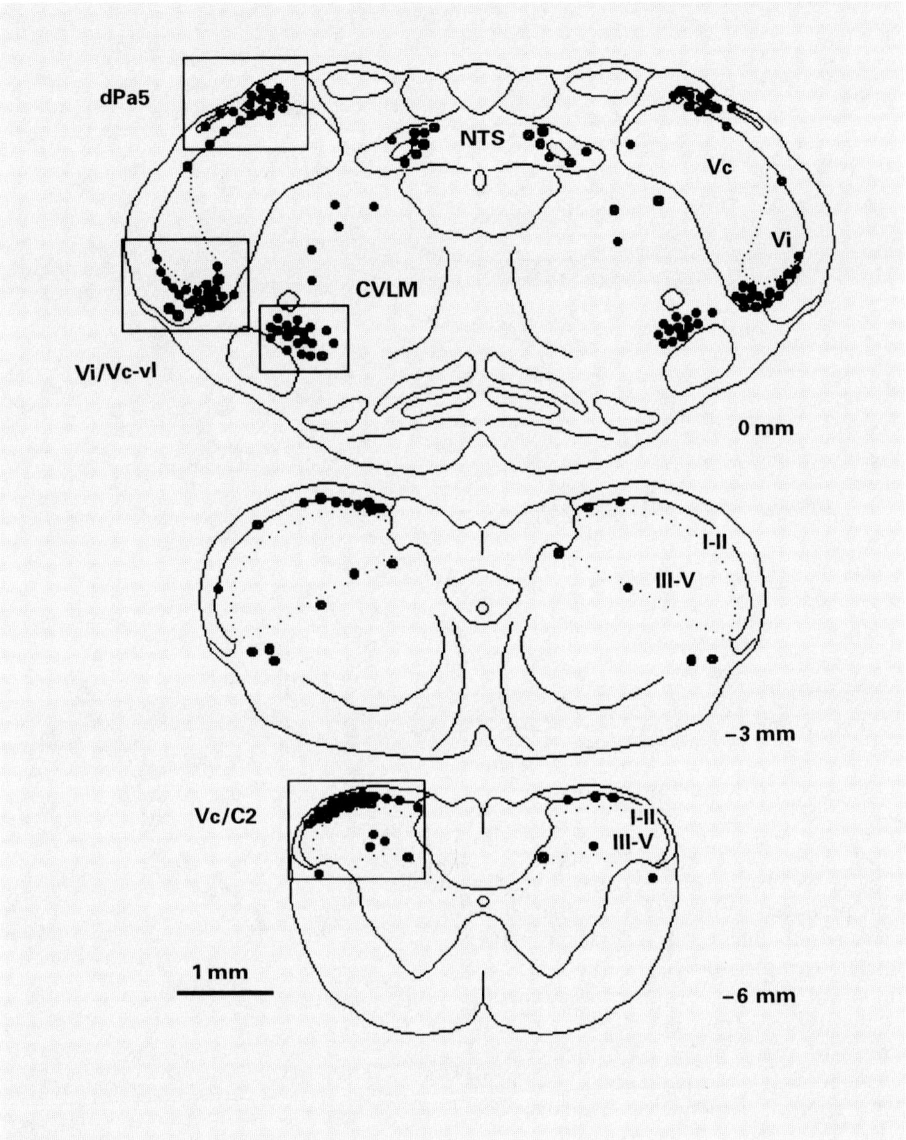

Fig. 2. An example of the pattern of Fos-positive neurons produced in one animal after injection of mustard oil (20% solution, 25 µl) drawn onto a series of camera lucida outlines. One dot = 1 Fos-positive neuron. The four boxes indicate the regions of high density of Fos-positive neurons that were compared statistically. dPa5 = Dorsal paratrigeminal nucleus; CVLM = caudal ventrolateral medulla; NTS = n. tractus solitarii; Vc = subnucleus caudalis; Vi = subnucleus interpolaris; I-II, III-V = laminae of Vc and upper cervical dorsal horn. Numbers to the right of each outline refer to the distance from the obex in mm.

morphine were given prior to 20% mustard oil injection into the TMJ region. Compared to the response to 20% mustard oil alone morphine pretreatment caused a dose-related reduction in Fos-LI at the dPa5 region of males and females (fig. 4, upper panel). In addition, high doses of morphine (3 and 7 mg/kg) caused a greater reduction in males than proestrus or diestrus females ($p < 0.01$). Morphine reduced Fos-LI at the Vi/Vc-vl transition region (fig. 4, middle panel) only after high doses (3 or 7 mg/kg) and was similar for males and females. At the Vc/C2 junction region (fig. 4, lower panel) morphine caused a significant dose-related reduction in Fos-positive neurons in males and females. In addition, as seen at the dPa5, the highest dose of morphine had a greater effect in males than females ($p < 0.05$). Naloxone reversed completely the inhibitory effect of morphine at each of these brainstem regions in males indicating a receptor-mediated mechanism, while in proestrus females naloxone partially prevented the effects of morphine. Animals that received morphine alone without TMJ injury displayed a similar number of Fos-positive neurons as drug-free unstimulated controls (data not shown).

Effect of U50,488H on Fos-LI in Specific Neuronal Cell Groups

To determine if kappa opioid mechanisms affected c-*fos* expression similarly in females and males, different doses of the selective kappa opioid receptor agonist, U50,488H, were given prior to 20% mustard oil injection into the TMJ region. In general, pretreatment with U50,488H had a more restricted effect on Fos-LI than morphine. At the dPa5 region U50,488H caused a significant dose-related reduction in Fos-LI only in proestrus females (fig. 5, upper panel). Diestrus females also displayed a small (though significant overall, $p < 0.05$) decrease while the number of Fos-positive neurons produced in dPa5 of males was not affected by U50,488H. At the Vi/Vc-vl transition region (fig. 5, middle panel), U50,488H had no significant effect on Fos-LI produced in females or males. By contrast, at the Vc/C2 junction region (fig. 5, lower panel), U50,488H caused a significant dose-related reduction in Fos-positive neurons in proestrus females, a small reduction in diestrus females and no effect in males. Note that in males a moderate dose of U50,488H (0.3 mg/kg) produced an increase in Fos-positive cells at the Vc/C2 junction region compared to TMJ injury alone ($p < 0.05$). The highest dose of U50,488H (7 mg/kg) caused a greater reduction in Fos-LI in proestrus females than diestrus females or males ($p < 0.01$). The selective kappa receptor antagonist, nor-BNI (16 mg/kg), only partially reversed the effect of U50,488H at the Vc/C2 junction region in proestrus females but had little or no effect on Fos-LI produced at dPa5 or the Vi/Vc-vl transition regions. High dose U50,488H alone (7 mg/kg) did not affect Fos-LI in any brainstem region compared to drug-free unstimulated controls (data not shown).

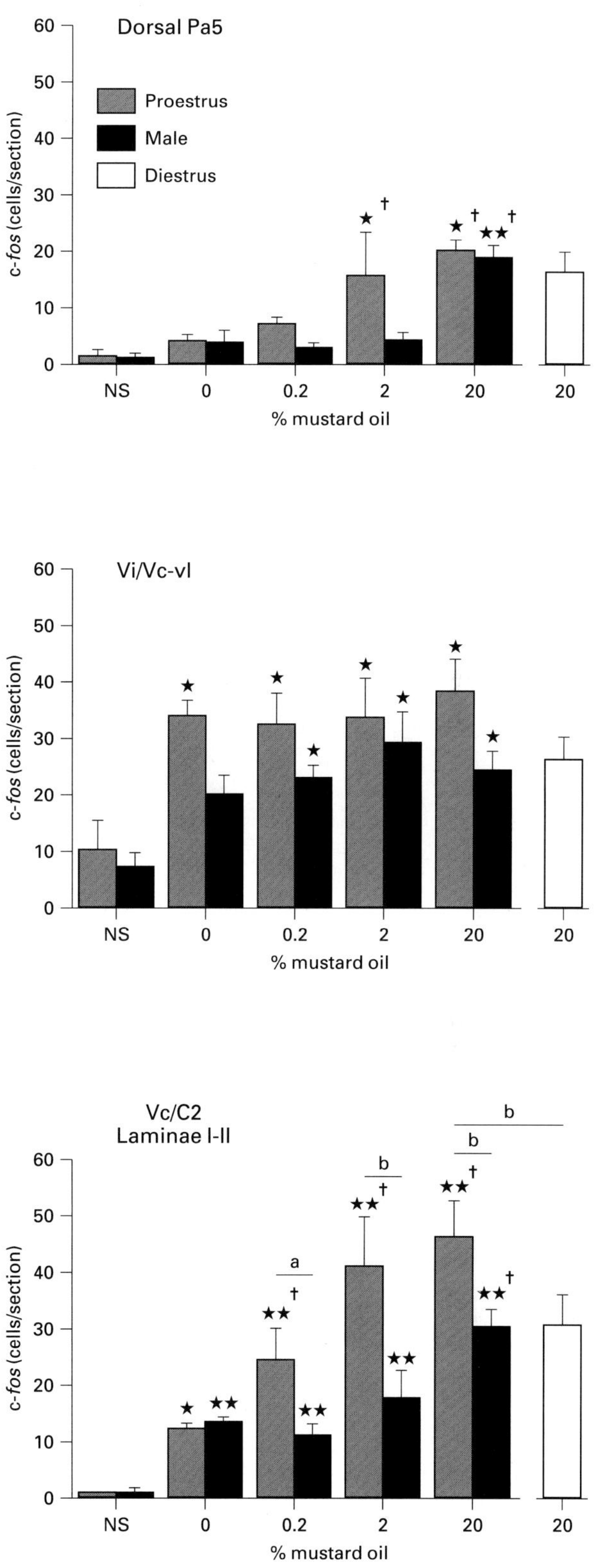

Fig. 3. Mean number of Fos-positive neurons produced in the dorsal paratrigeminal region (dPa5, top panel), trigeminal subnucleus interpolaris/caudalis transition region (Vi/Vc-vl, middle panel), and subnucleus caudalis/upper cervical cord junction (Vc/C2, lower panel) of proestrus females and males. Results indicate number of cells produced in unstimulated controls (left side) or ipsilateral to mustard oil injection (0.2–20%, 25 μl) into the TMJ region. For comparison the response of diestrus females to injection of 20% mustard oil is shown to the right of each panel (open bars). See boxed areas in figure 2 for regions of interest. NS = Unstimulated controls; 0 = saline injection; 0.2–20% = concentration of mustard oil; * $p < 0.05$, ** $p < 0.01$ versus unstimulated controls; † $p < 0.05$ vs. 0% mustard oil group; [a] $p < 0.05$, [b] $p < 0.01$ between animal groups.

4

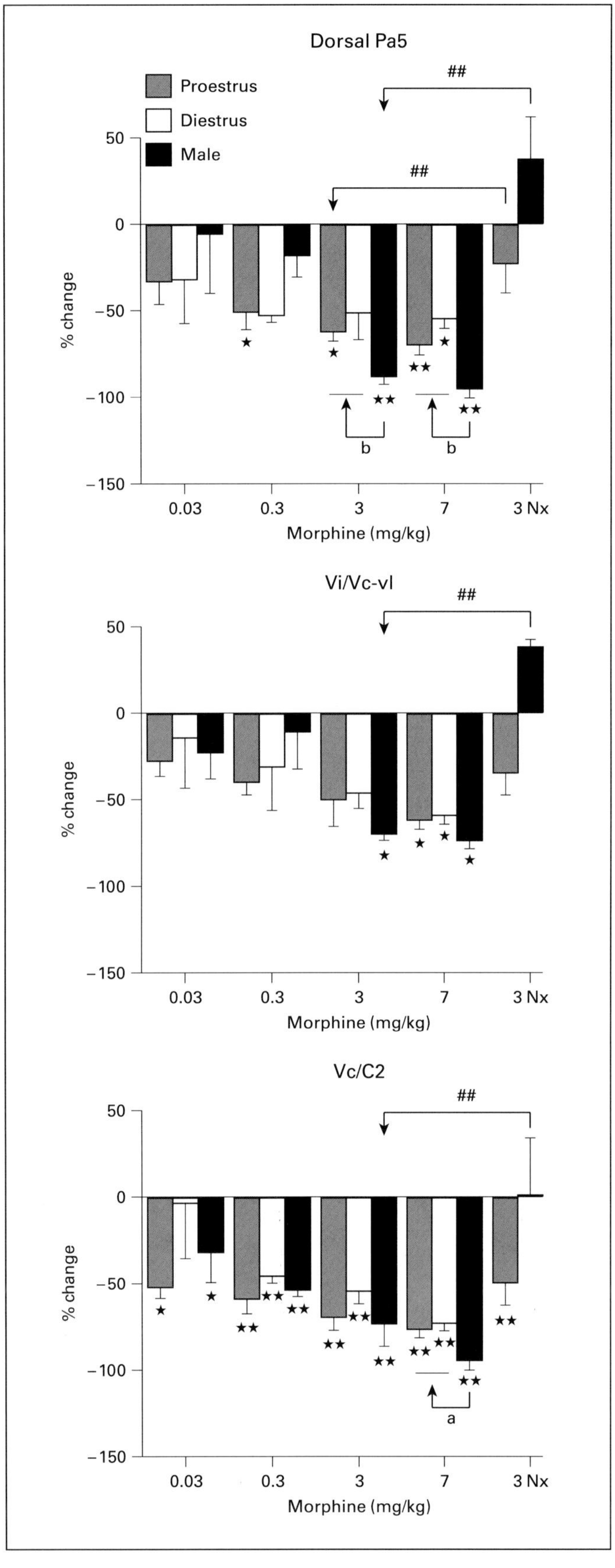
Dorsal Pa5
Proestrus
Diestrus
Male
##
##
50
0
−50
−100
−150
% change
b
b
0.03
0.3
3
7
3 Nx
Morphine (mg/kg)
Vi/Vc-vl
##
Morphine (mg/kg)
Vc/C2
##
a
Morphine (mg/kg)

5

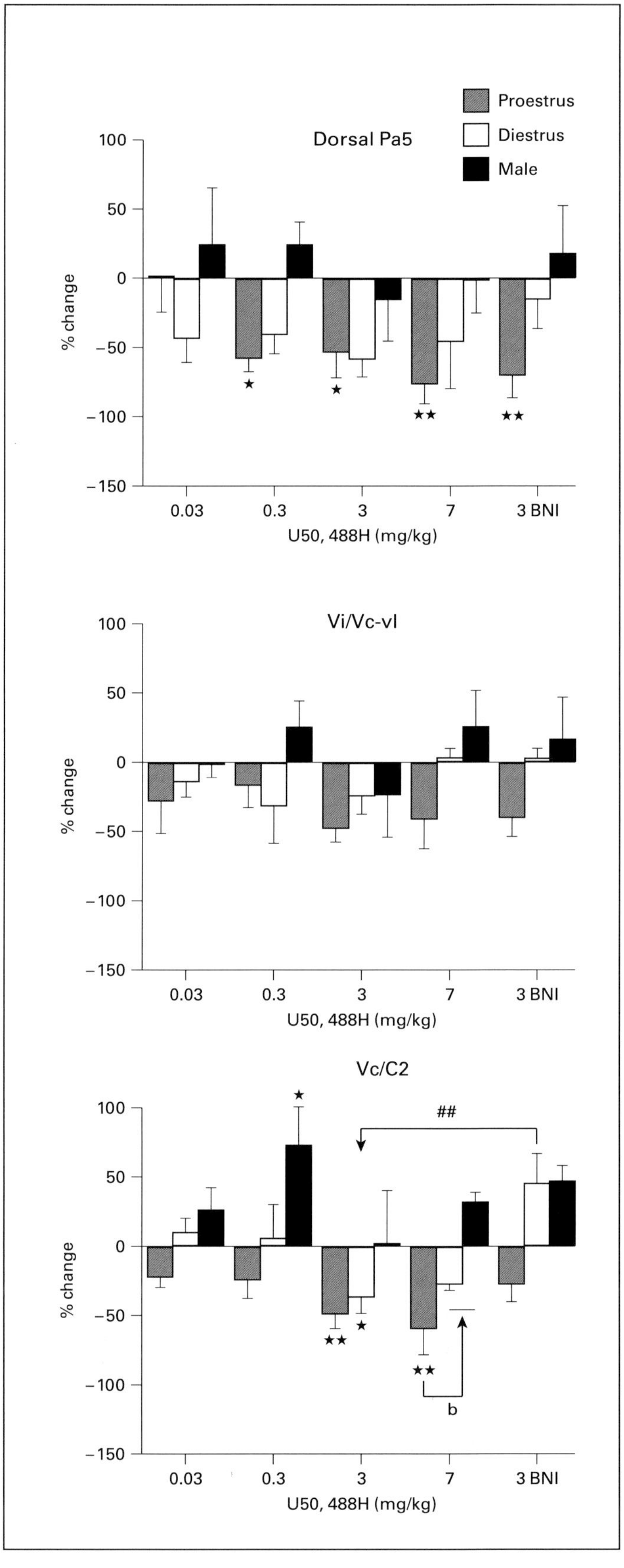
Proestrus
Diestrus
Male
Dorsal Pa5
100
50
0
−50
−100
−150
% change
0.03
0.3
3
7
3 BNI
U50, 488H (mg/kg)
Vi/Vc-vl
U50, 488H (mg/kg)
Vc/C2
##
b
U50, 488H (mg/kg)

Fos-LI in the Caudal Ventrolateral Medulla (CVLM)

The CVLM displayed a significant number of Fos-positive neurons bilaterally in all animal groups (see fig. 2). As shown in figure 6 (upper panel), unstimulated control proestrus females had higher levels of Fos-LI than males. Fos-LI increased significantly in proestrus females and males after TMJ injury independent of the concentration of mustard oil. Morphine pretreatment caused a moderate and similar dose-related reduction in Fos-LI in females and males compared to animals that received 20% mustard oil injection alone (fig. 6, lower panel). Pretreatment with U50,488H did not reduce the number of Fos-positive neurons compared to 20% mustard oil alone (data not shown).

Plasma extravasation as measured by Evan's blue dye extracted from muscle tissue adjacent to the TMJ region was similar for proestrus females and males (6.4 ± 1.2 vs. 6.9 ± 1.4 μg/g wet weight). Mean arterial pressure (MAP) averaged 123 ± 2, 112 ± 8 and 110 ± 7 mm Hg in proestrus females, diestrus females and males, respectively prior to TMJ injury. Injection of 20% mustard oil into the TMJ region caused a prompt and similar peak increase in MAP (>10 mm Hg) in males and females. Heart rate averaged 348 ± 22, 349 ± 16 and 380 ± 22 beats/min in proestrus females, diestrus females and males, respectively, prior to TMJ injury. Injection of 20% mustard oil caused a similar peak increase in heart rate (>10 beats per min) in males and females. The average body weights of males and females were not different.

Fig. 4. Effect of morphine on Fos-positive neurons produced in the dorsal paratrigeminal region (dPa5, top panel), trigeminal subnucleus interpolaris/caudalis transition region (Vi/Vc-vl, middle panel), and subnucleus caudalis/upper cervical cord junction (Vc/C2, lower panel) expressed as percentage change from the response to 20% mustard oil injection into the TMJ region. 3Nx = Morphine (3 mg/kg) plus naloxone (1 mg/kg i.v.); 0.3–7 = dose of morphine sulfate (mg/kg i.v.) given 10 min prior to TMJ injury. * $p < 0.05$, ** $p < 0.01$ vs. 20% mustard oil group; [a] $p < 0.05$, [b] $p < 0.01$ between animal groups; ## $p < 0.01$ vs. morphine plus naloxone.

Fig. 5. Effect of the kappa opioid receptor agonist, U50,488H, on Fos-positive neurons produced in the dorsal paratrigeminal region (dPa5, top panel), trigeminal subnucleus interpolaris/caudalis transition region (Vi/Vc-vl, middle panel), and subnucleus caudalis/upper cervical cord junction (Vc/C2, lower panel) expressed as percentage change from the response to 20% mustard oil injection into the TMJ region. 3BNI = U50,488H (3 mg/kg) plus nor-BNI (16 mg/kg i.v.); 0.3–7 = dose of U50,488H (mg/kg i.v.) given 10 min prior to TMJ injury. * $p < 0.05$, ** $p < 0.01$ vs. 20% mustard oil group; [a] $p < 0.05$, between animal groups; ## $p < 0.01$ vs. U50,488H plus nor-BNI.

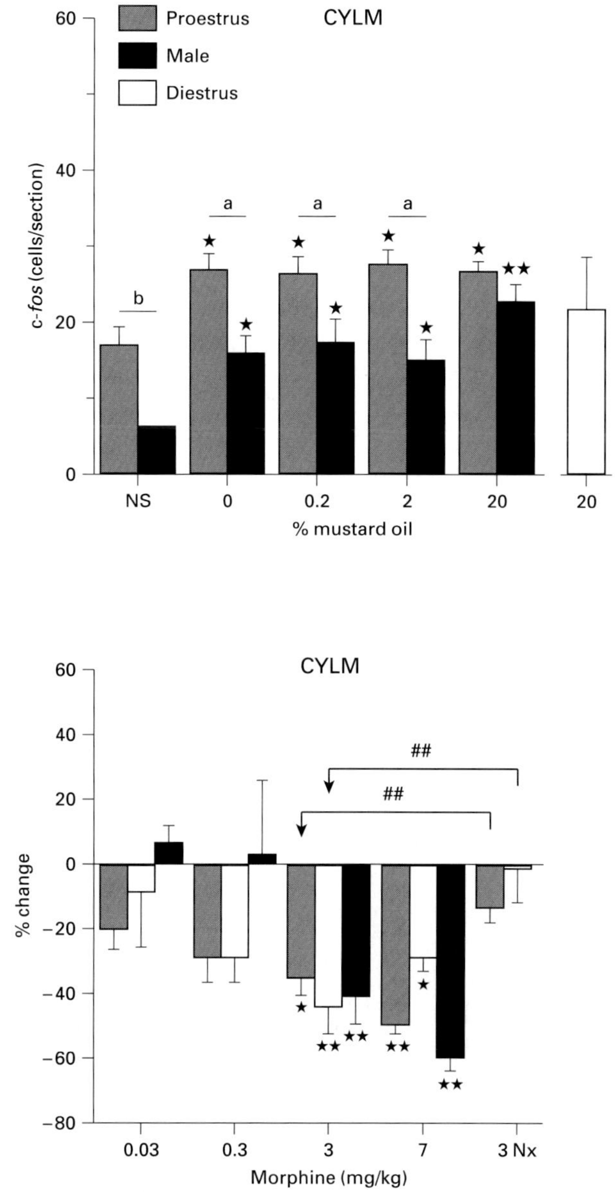

Fig. 6. Mean number of Fos-positive neurons produced in the caudal ventrolateral medulla (CVLM) in unstimulated controls or ipsilateral to mustard oil injection (0.2–20%, 25 μl) into the TMJ region of proestrus females and males (upper panel). For comparison the response of diestrus females to injection of 20% mustard oil is shown to the right of each panel (open bars). See boxed area in figure 2 for region of interest. Lower panel indicates the effect of morphine pretreatment on the number of cells produced in CVLM expressed as percentage change from the response to 20% mustard oil injection into the TMJ region. NS = Unstimulated controls; 0 = saline injection into TMJ region; 0.2–20% = concentration of mustard oil. * $p < 0.05$, ** $p < 0.01$ vs. unstimulated controls; [a] $p < 0.05$, [b] $p < 0.01$ between animal groups; ## $p < 0.01$ versus morphine plus naloxone.

Discussion

Although women have a higher prevalence of TMD pain than men [LeResche, 1997], the basis for this finding remains uncertain [Stohler, 1997]. To test the hypothesis that neurobiological mechanisms underlie such sex differences and occur at the initial stages of integration within the CNS, Fos, the protein product of the immediate early gene, c-*fos* was quantified in males and females after TMJ injury. The results indicated that TMJ injury produced a greater number of Fos-positive neurons in the trigeminal brainstem complex and upper cervical dorsal horn of proestrus females than diestrus females or males. In addition, opioid modulation of Fos-LI produced by TMJ injury displayed significant sex differences. Morphine caused a greater inhibition of Fos-LI in males compared to proestrus or diestrus females, while the selective kappa opioid receptor agonist, U50,488H, caused consistent dose-related reductions in Fos-LI after TMJ injury only in proestrus females.

Fos-LI as a Marker for Primary Afferent Input from the TMJ Region

As reported previously [Hathaway et al., 1995; Bereiter and Bereiter, 2000], acute inflammation of the TMJ region produced Fos-LI in three spatially distinct regions of the trigeminal spinal nucleus: dPa5, Vi/Vc-vl transition region, and laminae I-II at the Vc/C2 junction region. Comparisons with the distribution of central terminals seen after transganglionic labeling of trigeminal [Jacquin et al., 1983; Takemura et al., 1987], upper cervical [Pfaller and Arvidsson, 1988; Neuhuber and Zenker, 1989], or vagal afferent nerves [Contreras et al., 1982], suggested a high percentage of Fos-positive neurons produced at the dPa5 and Vc/C2 junction region resulted from direct input from primary afferent fibers. By contrast, Fos-LI produced at the Vi/Vc-vl transition region more likely represented third- or higher-order neurons since few primary afferent fibers project from the TMJ region to this brainstem area. Fos-positive neurons produced at the Vi/Vc-vl transition region may have been due to the relay of nociceptor input from the Vc/C2 junction region via intratrigeminal connections. Recent electrophysiological studies have revealed direct connections from the caudal portions of Vc to the Vi/Vc-vl transition region that could contribute to the processing of corneal sensory information [Hirata et al., 2000].

Sex Differences and Fos-LI Produced after TMJ Injury

Although the exact relationship between the sex of the animal and activity of brainstem neurons cannot be determined by this approach alone, both peripheral and central mechanisms could contribute to the sex differences in Fos-LI seen after TMJ injury. Levels of Fos-LI varied over the estrous cycle suggesting that circulating factors such as sex steroids contributed to these results. Sex steroids could act peripherally to enhance the magnitude of the pain signal or number of nociceptors excited by TMJ injury in proestrus females relative to males. A peripheral site of action for sex steroids is supported by studies in which acute exposure to estrogen elevated the content of calcitonin gene-related peptide (CGRP) levels in spinal dorsal root ganglion (DRG) cells [Gangula et al., 2000]. CGRP is a nociceptive neuropeptide contained in many TMJ primary afferent fibers [Kido et al., 1993; Uddman et al., 1998]. Similarly, estrogen rapidly increased the expression of nerve growth factor receptor mRNA in spinal DRGs [Sohrabji et al., 1994]. An estrogen-nerve growth factor link has been proposed as a possible risk factor in TMD pain [Stohler, 1997]. Single unit recording studies have demonstrated that the receptive field size of trigeminal ganglion neurons can vary during the estrous cycle [Bereiter and Barker, 1980]; however, the properties of nociceptive trigeminal ganglion cells were not determined. Sex steroids could affect the inflammatory response caused by mustard oil and thus, indirectly, alter the activity of TMJ nociceptors by modifying the levels of inflammatory agents released into the injured region. However, in a recent study in which bradykinin was injected into the knee joint, plasma extravasation was shown to be greater in male than female rats, a sex differences that was prevented by ovariectomy and restored by estrogen [Green et al., 1999].

Sex steroids also could act centrally to modify Fos-LI production after TMJ injury. Thus, pain signals arising from peripheral TMJ nociceptors could be similar in males and females, but are processed differently within the brain. Estrogen receptors (ER) are found throughout the CNS including the superficial laminae of the Vc/C2 junction region [Shughrue et al., 1997], the brainstem region that displayed the greatest sex differences in number of Fos-positive neurons produced after TMJ injury (fig. 3). More than 40% of ER-positive neurons found in laminae I-II at the Vc/C2 junction region colocalized preproenkephalin mRNA [Amandusson et al., 1996], whereas in lower levels of spinal dorsal horn more than 80% of Fos-positive neurons seen after acute inflammation also expressed preproenkephalin mRNA [Noguchi et al., 1992]. These results suggested that Fos-positive neurons in the superficial laminae of the medullary and spinal dorsal horns may regulate endogenous opioid peptide formation in local circuits. ER-positive neurons also are found in significant numbers in the periaqueductal gray of female rats [Shugrue et al., 1997], a pontine region well associated with opioid analgesia and descending pain control pathways [Fields and Basbaum, 1994]. Considerable evidence indicates that exogenous opioids have differential effects on pain behavior in male and female animals [Cicero et al., 1997; Kest et al., 2000], including studies in which opioid drugs are microinjected directly into the periaqueductal gray area [Krzanowska and Bodnar, 1999]

The present results indicated that morphine caused dose-related decreases in Fos-LI at the dPa5 and Vc/C2 junction region that were greater in males than proestrus females in agreement with the magnitude of exogenous morphine on pain behavior in males and females [Cicero et al., 1997; Krzanowska and Bodnar, 1999; Kest et al., 2000]. The magnitude of morphine-induced inhibition of Fos-LI also agreed with the relative density of mu opioid receptors in these brainstem regions [Ding et al., 1996]. However, it is not yet certain if the properties and/or density of opioid receptors are similar for males and females in the trigeminal complex or supraspinal pain control regions such as the periaqueductal gray. Compared to the widespread effect of morphine in which Fos-LI was reduced in males as well as females at the dPa5, Vi/Vc-vl transition and Vc/C2 junction regions, U50,488H caused a significant dose-related reduction in Fos-LI only at the dPa5 and Vc/C2 transition region and only in proestrus females. These results were consistent with recent evidence that kappa opioid receptor density in the lumbar dorsal horn cord varied during the estrous cycle with the highest density occurring during proestrus [Chang et al., 2000]. Unexpectedly, U50,488H did not reduce the number of Fos-positive neurons in any trigeminal brainstem region in males despite anatomical evidence for moderate levels of kappa opioid receptors in the medullary and spinal dorsal horns [Mansour et al., 1996]. These results also contrast with previous studies in which kappa opioid agonists prevented an increase in Fos-LI after acute inflammation of cutaneous [Catheline et al., 1999] or visceral [Hammond et al., 1992] tissues in male rats. In human studies kappa opioids provided longer relief from dental pain in females than males [Gear et al., 1996]. In male monkeys U50,488H reduced cutaneous thermal sensitivity more than in ovariectomized females, although estrogen replacement therapy enhanced the effectiveness of kappa opioids on pain behavior in females but not in males [Negus and Mello, 1999]. These apparently conflicting results support suggestions [Bartok and Craft, 1997; Kest et al., 2000] that the nature and/or source of the pain signal determine the relative effectiveness of different classes of opioid drugs in males and females.

Psychophysical studies indicate that a central neural dysfunction, such as an altered ability to recruit endogenous pain control pathways, may cause TMD pain in some patients. TMD patients displayed enhanced temporal summation of thermal pain and enhanced C-fiber summation compared to pain free controls [Maixner et al., 1998]. In control subjects submaximal tourniquet stress caused an elevation in the time to ischemic pain tolerance that was reversed by naloxone. However, in TMD patients tourniquet stress did not reduce TMD pain and naloxone did not shorten the time to ischemic pain tolerance suggesting that the normal recruitment of endogenous opioid mechanisms was deficient in these patients [Maixner et al., 1995b]. It remains to be determined if the ability to recruit endogenous pain control pathways is similar and under which conditions might this ability differs for males and females.

Fos-Positive Neurons and Different Aspects of TMD Pain

Acute injury to the TMJ region produced Fos-LI in several spatially discrete regions of the caudal brainstem complex and upper cervical spinal cord. Although c-*fos* immunocytochemistry cannot reveal the exact function of neurons in these regions, these results suggested the dPa5, Vi/Vc-vl transition and Vc/C2 junction regions mediated different aspects of TMD pain. Mustard oil dose-effect relationships suggested that Fos-LI produced at the Vc/C2 junction region, and to a lesser extent in the dPa5 region, encoded the intensity of the inflammatory stimulus. Since morphine (males and females) and U50,488H (proestrus females only) also had the greatest inhibitory effect on Fos-LI produced in the Vc/C2 junction region, a region with connections to the sensory thalamus [Carstens et al., 1990] it is proposed that cells in this region mediate the sensory-discriminative aspects of TMD pain. By contrast, Fos-LI produced in the Vi/Vc-vl transition region did not encode the intensity of the inflammatory stimulus, but rather displayed a similar dose-effect relationship as the CVLM region, and revealed only a moderate reduction after morphine and no reduction after U50,488H. Since the Vi/Vc-vl transition region is unique among caudal trigeminal brainstem regions with a high density of efferent projections to thalamic nucleus submedius [Yoshida et al., 1991], it is proposed that the Vi/Vc-vl neurons may function to recruit endogenous pain control mechanisms. The enhanced Fos-LI seen within the CVLM of proestrus females supports the notion of an autonomic nervous system component in TMD pain [Maixner et al., 1995b].

In summary, acute inflammatory injury of the TMJ region activated several spatially distinct regions of the trigeminal spinal nucleus and upper cervical dorsal horn as seen by an increase in the number Fos-positive neurons. Although the pattern of Fos-LI was similar in males and females, the magnitude of expression and its modulation by opioid receptor agonists revealed significant sex-related differences. Based on the responses to different intensities of inflammation and differential sensitivity to opioid analgesics, these results support the conclusion that second-order neurons in laminae I-II at the Vc/C2 junction region play a critical role in mediating sex differences related to TMD pain.

Acknowledgements

The author thanks D.F. Bereiter and A. Pooler for excellent technical support and Dr. Harumitsu Hirata for helpful comments in preparing the manuscript. This study was supported by a grant from the NIDCR (DE-12758).

References

Amandusson, A., O. Hermanson, A. Blomqvist (1996) Colocalization of oestrogen receptor immunoreactivity and preproenkephalin mRNA expression to neurons in the superficial laminae of the spinal and medullary dorsal horn of rats. Eur J Neurosci *8:* 2440–2445.

Bartok, R.E., R.M. Craft (1997) Sex differences in opioid antinociception. J Pharmacol Exp Ther *282:* 769–778.

Bereiter, D.A. (1997) Morphine and somatostatin analogue reduce c-*fos* expression in trigeminal subnucleus caudalis produced by corneal stimulation in the rat. Neuroscience *77:* 864–874.

Bereiter, D.A., D.J. Barker (1980) Hormone-induced enlargement of receptive fields in trigeminal mechanoreceptive neurons. I. Time course, hormone, sex and modality specificity. Brain Res *184:* 395–410.

Bereiter, D.A., D.F. Bereiter (2000) Morphine and NMDA receptor antagonism reduced c-*fos* expression in spinal trigeminal nucleus produced by acute injury to the TMJ region. Pain *85:* 65–77.

Bullitt, E. (1990) Expression of c-*fos*-like protein as a marker for neuronal activity following noxious stimulation in the rat. J Comp Neurol *296:* 517–530.

Carstens, E., J. Leah, J. Lechner, M. Zimmermann (1990) Demonstration of extensive brainstem connections to medial and lateral thalamus and hypothalamus in the rat. Neuroscience *35:* 609–626.

Catheline, G., S.L. Guen, J.-M. Besson (1999) Effects of U-69,593, a k-opioid receptor agonist, on carrageenin-induced peripheral oedema and Fos expression in the rat spinal cord. Eur J Pharmacol *370:* 287–296.

Chang, P.C., S.A. Aicher, C. Drake (2000) Kappa opioid receptors in rat spinal cord vary across the estrous cycle. Brain Res *861:* 168–172.

Cicero, T.J., B. Nock, E.R. Meyer (1997) Sex-related differences in morphine's antinociceptive activity: Relationship to serum and brain morphine concentrations. J Pharmacol Exp Ther *282:* 939–944.

Contreras, R.J., R.M. Beckstead, R. Norgren (1982) The central projections of the trigeminal, facial, glossopharyngeal and vagus nerves: An autoradiographic study in the rat. J Auton Nerv Syst *6:* 303–322.

Dampney, R.A.L. (1994) Functional organization of central pathways regulating the cardiovascular system. Physiol Rev *74:* 323–364.

Denny-Brown, D., N. Yanagisawa (1973) The function of the descending root of the fifth nerve. Brain *96:* 783–814.

Ding, Y.-Q., T. Kaneko, S. Nomura, N. Mizuno (1996) Immunohistochemical localization of μ-opioid receptors in the central nervous system of the rat. J Comp Neurol *367:* 375–402.

Fields, H., A.I. Basbaum (1994) Central nervous sysem mechanisms of pain modulation; in Wall P.D., R. Melzack (eds): Textbook of Pain. Edinburgh, Churchill Livingstone, pp 243–257.

Gangula, P.R., P. Lanlua, S. Wimalawansa, S. Supowit, D. DiPette, C. Yallampalli (2000) Regulation of calcitonin gene-related peptide expression in dorsal root ganglia of rats by female sex steroid hormones. Biol Reprod *62:* 1033–1039.

Gear, R.W., C. Miaskowski, N.C. Gordon, S.M. Paul, P.H. Heller, J.D. Levine (1996) Kappa-opioids produce significantly greater analgesia in women than in men. Nat Med *2:* 1248–1250.

Green, P.G., S.R. Dahlqvist, W.M. Isenberg, H.J. Strausbaugh, F.J. Miao, J.D. Levine (1999) Sex steroid regulation of the inflammatory response: Sympathoadrenal dependence in the female rat. J Neurosci *19:* 4082–4089.

Haas, D.A., O. Nakanishi, R.E. MacMillan, R.C. Jordan, J.W. Hu (1992) Development of an orofacial model of acute inflammation in the rat. Arch Oral Biol *37:* 417–422.

Hammond, D.L., R. Presley, K.R. Gogas, A.I. Basbaum (1992) Morphine or U-50,488 suppresses Fos protein-like immunoreactivity in the spinal cord and nucleus tractus solitarii evoked by a noxious visceral stimulus in the rat. J Comp Neurol *315:* 244–253.

Hathaway, C.B., J.W. Hu, D.A. Bereiter (1995) Distribution of Fos-like immunoreactivity in the caudal brainstem of the rat following noxious chemical stimulation of the temporomandibular joint. J Comp Neurol *356:* 444–456.

Hirata, H., S. Takeshita, J.W. Hu, D.A. Bereiter (2000) Cornea-responsive medullary dorsal horn neurons: Modulation by local opioid agonists and projections to thalamus and brainstem. J Neurophysiol *84:* 1050–1061.

Hunt, S.P., A. Pini, G. Evan (1987) Induction of c-*fos*-like protein in spinal cord neurons following sensory stimulation. Nature *328:* 632–634.

Jacquin, M.F., K. Semba, M.D. Egger, R.W. Rhoades (1983) Organization of HRP-labeled trigeminal mandibular primary afferent neurons in the rat. J Comp Neurol *215:* 397–420.

Kest, B., E. Sarton, A. Dahan (2000) Gender differences in opioid-mediated analgesia: Animal and human studies. Anesthesiology *9:* 539–547.

Kido, M.A., T. Kiyoshima, T. Kondo, N. Ayasaka, R. Moroi, Y. Terada, T. Tanaka (1993) Distribution of substance P and calcitonin gene-related peptide-like immunoreactive nerve fibers in the rat temporomandibular joint. J Dent Res *72:* 592–598.

Klineberg, I. (1971) Structure and function of temporomandibular joint innervation. Ann Roy Coll Surg Engl *49:* 268–288.

Krzanowska, E.K., R.J. Bodnar (1999) Morphine antinociception elicited from the ventrolateral periaqueductal gray is sensitive to sex and gonadectomy differences in rats. Brain Res *821:* 224–230.

LeResche, L. (1997) Epidemiology of temporomandibular disorders: Implications for the investigation of etiological factors. Crit Rev Oral Biol Med *8:* 291–305.

LeResche, L., K. Saunders, M.R.V. Korff, W. Barlow, S.F. Dworkin (1997) Use of exogenous hormones and risk of temporomandibular disorder pain. Pain *69:* 153–160.

Lu, J., C.B. Hathaway, D.A. Bereiter (1993) Adrenalectomy enhances Fos-like immunoreactivity within the spinal trigeminal nucleus induced by noxious thermal stimulation of the cornea. Neuroscience *54:* 809–818.

Maixner, W., R. Fillingim, D. Booker, A. Sigurdsson (1995a) Sensitivity of patients with painful temporomandibular disorders to experimentally evoked pain. Pain *63:* 341–351.

Maixner, W., R. Fillingim, A. Sigurdsson, S. Kincaid, S. Silva (1998) Sensitivity of patients with temporomandibular disorders to experimentally evoked pain: Evidence for altered temporal summation of pain. Pain *76:* 71–81.

Maixner, W., A. Sigurdsson, R.B. Fillingim, T. Lundeen, D.K. Booker (1995b) Regulation of acute and chronic orofacial pain; in Fricton J.R., R. Dubner (eds): Orofacial Pain and Temporomandibular Disorders. New York, Raven Press, pp 85–102.

Mansour, A., S. Burke, R.J. Pavlic, H. Akil, S.J. Watson (1996) Immunohistochemical localization of the cloned kappa-1 receptor in the rat CNS and pituitary. Neuroscience *71:* 671–690.

Meng, I.D., D.A. Bereiter (1996) Differential distribution of Fos-like immunoreactivity in the spinal trigeminal nucleus after noxious and innocuous thermal and chemical stimulation of rat cornea. Neuroscience *72:* 243–254.

Molander, C., Q. Xu, C. Rivero-Melian, G. Grant (1989) Cytoarchitectonic organization of the spinal cord in the rat: II. The cervical and upper thoracic cord. J Comp Neurol *289:* 375–385.

Negus, S.S., N.K. Mello (1999) Opioid antinociception in ovariectomized monkeys: Comparison with antinociception in males and effects of estradiol replacement. J Pharmacol Exp Ther *290:* 1132–1140.

Neuhuber, W.L., W. Zenker (1989) Central distribution of cervical primary afferents in the rat, with emphasis on proprioceptive projections to vestibular, perihypoglossal, and upper thoracic spinal nuclei. J Comp Neurol *280:* 231–253.

Noguchi, K., R. Dubner, M.A. Ruda (1992) Preproenkephalin mRNA in spinal dorsal horn neurons is induced by peripheral inflammation and is co-localized with Fos and Fos-related proteins. Neuroscience *46:* 561–570.

Pfaller, K., J. Arvidsson (1988) Central distribution of trigeminal and upper cervical primary afferents in the rat studied by anterograde transport of horseradish peroxidase conjugated to wheat germ agglutinin. J Comp Neurol *268:* 91–108.

Presley, R.W., D. Menetrey, J.D. Levine, A.I. Basbaum (1990) Systemic morphine suppresses noxious stimulus-evoked fos protein-like immunoreactivity in the rat spinal cord. J Neurosci *10:* 323–335.

Shughrue, P.J., M.V. Lane, I. Merchenthaler (1997) Comparative distribution of estrogen receptor-a and -b mRNA in the rat central nervous system. J Comp Neurol *388:* 507–525.

Sohrabji, F., R.C. Miranda, C.D. Toran-Allerand (1994) Estrogen differentially regulates estrogen and nerve growth factor receptor mRNAs in adult sensory neurons. J Neurosci *14:* 459–471.

Stohler, C.S. (1995) Clinical perspectives on masticatory and related muscle disorders; in Sessle, B.J., P.S. Bryant, R.A. Dionne (eds): Temporomandibular Disorders and Related Pain Conditions. Seattle, IASP, pp 3–29.

Stohler, C.S. (1997) Masticatory myalgias: Emphasis on the nerve growth factor-estrogen link. Pain Forum *6:* 176–180.

Strassman, A.M., B.P. Vos (1993) Somatotopic and laminar organization of Fos-like immunoreactivity in the medullary and cervical dorsal horn induced by noxious facial stimulation in the rat. J Comp Neurol *331:* 495–516.

Takemura, M., T. Sugimoto, A. Sakai (1987) Topographic organization of central terminal region of different sensory branches of the rat mandibular nerve. Exp Neurol *96:* 540–557.

Uddman, R., T. Grunditz, J. Kato, F. Sundler (1998) Distribution and origin of nerve fibers in the rat temporomandibular joint capsule. Anat Embryol *197:* 273–282.

Widenfalk, B., M. Wiberg (1990) Origin of sympathetic and sensory innervation of the temporomandibular joint: A retrograde axonal tracing study in the rat. Neurosci Lett *109:* 30–35.

Winer, B.J. (1971) Statistical Principles in Experimental Design. New York, McGraw-Hill.

Yoshida, A., J.O. Dostrovsky, B.J. Sessle, C.Y. Chiang (1991) Trigeminal projections to the nucleus submedius of the thalamus in the rat. J Comp Neurol *307:* 609–625.

Cells Tissues Organs

Cells Tissues Organs 2001;169:238–247

Orofacial Deep and Cutaneous Tissue Inflammation and Trigeminal Neuronal Activation

Implications for Persistent Temporomandibular Pain

Hiroki Imbe[a] Koichi Iwata[b] Qi-Qi Zhou[a] Shiping Zou[a] Ronald Dubner[a] Ke Ren[a]

[a]Department of Oral and Craniofacial Biological Sciences, University of Maryland Dental School, Baltimore, Md., USA;
[b]Department of Oral Physiology, Faculty of Dentistry, Osaka University, Osaka, Japan

Key Words
Complete Freund's adjuvant · Fos protein · Preprodynorphin gene · Paratrigeminal nucleus · Evans' blue extravasation

Abstract
A rat model has been developed to characterize the responses of brainstem trigeminal neurons to orofacial deep and cutaneous tissue inflammation and hyperalgesia. Complete Freund's adjuvant (CFA) was injected unilaterally into the rat temporomandibular joint (TMJ) or perioral (PO) skin to produce inflammation in deep or cutaneous tissues, respectively. The TMJ and PO inflammation resulted in orofacial behavioral hyperalgesia and allodynia that peaked within 4–24 h and persisted for at least 2 weeks. Compared to cutaneous CFA injection, the injection of CFA into the TMJ produced a significantly stronger inflammation associated with a selective upregulation of preprodynorphin mRNA in the trigeminal spinal complex, an enhanced medullary dorsal horn hyperexcitability, and a greater trigeminal Fos protein expression, a marker of neuronal activation. The Fos-LI induced by TMJ inflammation persisted longer, was more intense, particularly in the superficial laminae, and more widespread rostrocaudally. Thus, the inflammatory irritant produces a stronger effect in deep than in cutaneous orofacial tissue. As there is heavy innervation of the TMJ by unmyelinated nerve endings, a strong nociceptive primary afferent barrage is expected following inflammation. An increase in TMJ C-fiber input after inflammation

Abbreviations used in this paper

CFA	complete Freund's adjuvant
HRP	horse radish peroxidase
HWL	head withdrawal latency
LI	like immunoreactivity
MDH	medullary dorsal horn
NS	nociceptive specific
Pa5	paratrigeminal nucleus
PO	perioral
PPD	preprodynorphin
PPE	preproenkephalin
RF	receptive field
TMJ	temporomandibular joint
Vc	subnucleus caudalis of the spinal trigeminal nucleus
Vi	subnucleus interpolaris of the spinal trigeminal nucleus
Vsp	spinal trigeminal nucleus
WDR	wide dynamic range

KARGER

Fax + 41 61 306 12 34
E-Mail karger@karger.ch
www.karger.com

Accessible online at:
www.karger.com/journals/cto

K. Ren, PhD
Department of OCBS
666 W, Baltimore St., Rm. 5A12
Baltimore, MD 21201 (USA)
Tel. +1 410 706 3250, Fax +1 410 706 4172, E-Mail kren@umaryland.edu

and strong central neuronal activation may initiate central hyperexcitability and contribute to persistent pain associated with temporomandibular disorders. Since deep inputs may be more effective in inducing central neuronal excitation than cutaneous inputs, greater sensory disturbances may occur in pain conditions involving deep tissues than in those involving cutaneous tissues.

Disorders of the temporomandibular joint (TMJ) and muscles of mastication often result in persistent pain and therefore are a major health problem. Women appear to be affected more than men [Carlsson and LeResche, 1995]. The underlying etiology and pathology associated with these disorders remains unclear. The development of animal models of tissue injury leading to pain and hyperalgesia has triggered major advances in our understanding of persistent pain of cutaneous origin [Dubner and Ren, 1999]. The lack of appropriate models for deep tissue pain, particularly in the orofacial region, has been a major deterrent to further understanding.

Most of our knowledge about mechanisms of persistent pain is based on studies of cutaneous pain in animals, experimental subjects and patients. Although it is tempting to generalize these findings to pain of deep tissues such as muscle and joint, there are important differences between cutaneous and deep pain [Dubner, 1991]. Cutaneous pain is highly localized to the site of stimulation and is described as sharp, stabbing or pricking. In contrast, deep pains are diffuse and difficult to localize and often described as aching and cramping. Another interesting clinical observation is that deep pains often refer to cutaneous sites whereas the reverse is rarely observed. Common to both cutaneous and deep persistent pains is the finding of increased sensitivity to painful stimuli and pain produced by innocuous stimulation. The peripheral and central nervous system mechanisms that underlie these phenomena need to be understood before new approaches to the treatment of muscle and joint pain can be developed.

Injection of inflammatory agents such as complete Freund's adjuvant (CFA) or carrageenan into the hindpaw of the rat produces an intense inflammation characterized by edema, redness and hyperalgesia that is limited to the injected paw and persists for days [Hargreaves et al., 1988; Iadarola et al., 1988a; Stein et al., 1988]. Since a variety of orofacial pain conditions also are associated with inflammation, including some forms of temporomandibular disorders [Shellhas et al., 1989], we have adapted this model to the orofacial region [Ren and Dubner, 1996; Imbe and Ren, 1999; Iwata et al., 1999; Ren, 1999; Zhou et al., 1999]. Following injection of CFA into the TMJ or perioral (PO) skin, rats developed persistent behavioral hyperalgesia associated with orofacial inflammation, resembling that seen in the hindpaw inflammation model. There was also a selective upregulation of opioid gene expression, the development of medullary dorsal horn hyperexcitability, and persistent Fos protein expression, a marker of neuronal activation, following orofacial deep and cutaneous tissue inflammation. We will briefly review these new findings and discuss their significance in persistent temporomandibular pain.

Behavioral Hyperalgesia

The injection of CFA or saline into the orofacial region appeared to have temporary non-specific effects on the animal's feeding behavior. The rats that received either CFA or saline injection stopped gaining weight for the first week (but no significant weight loss), as compared to noninjected naive rats. In the second week after inflammation, however, they started to gain weight and there was no significant difference in weight increases between the different groups of animals. Overall, the CFA-inflamed rats showed normal grooming behavior and levels of activity, indicating that the effect of inflammation and hyperalgesia on behavior of the animal was minimal. The CFA-induced inflammation was verified with Evan's blue dye (5 mg/kg i.v. 0.2%) extravasation. Postmortem examination of the injected TMJ region found accumulation of the blue dye in the TMJ and periarticular tissue, indicating plasma protein extravasation due to localized inflammation. This animal model has been approved by the Institutional Animal Care and Use Committee of the University of Maryland Dental School.

Orofacial thermal hyperalgesia was assessed by a method modified from Imamura et al. [1997]. A noxious thermal stimulus was directed to the skin above the TMJ and PO skin area and the head withdrawal latencies (HWL) were determined in lightly anesthetized rats (pentobarbital sodium, 20 mg/kg i.p.). A clear thermal hyperalgesia on the ipsilateral inflamed site was revealed. In TMJ-inflamed rats, ipsilateral HWL to stimulation of cutaneous tissues above the TMJ was reduced from 7.3 ± 0.8 to 5.0 ± 0.3 s (n = 7) 24 h following CFA injection (fig. 1A) (ANOVA, $F_{5,30} = 3.76$, $p < 0.01$). In PO skin-inflamed rats, ipsilateral HWL to PO stimulation was reduced from 7.1 ± 0.5 to 2.5 ± 0.1 s (n = 6) 24 h follow-

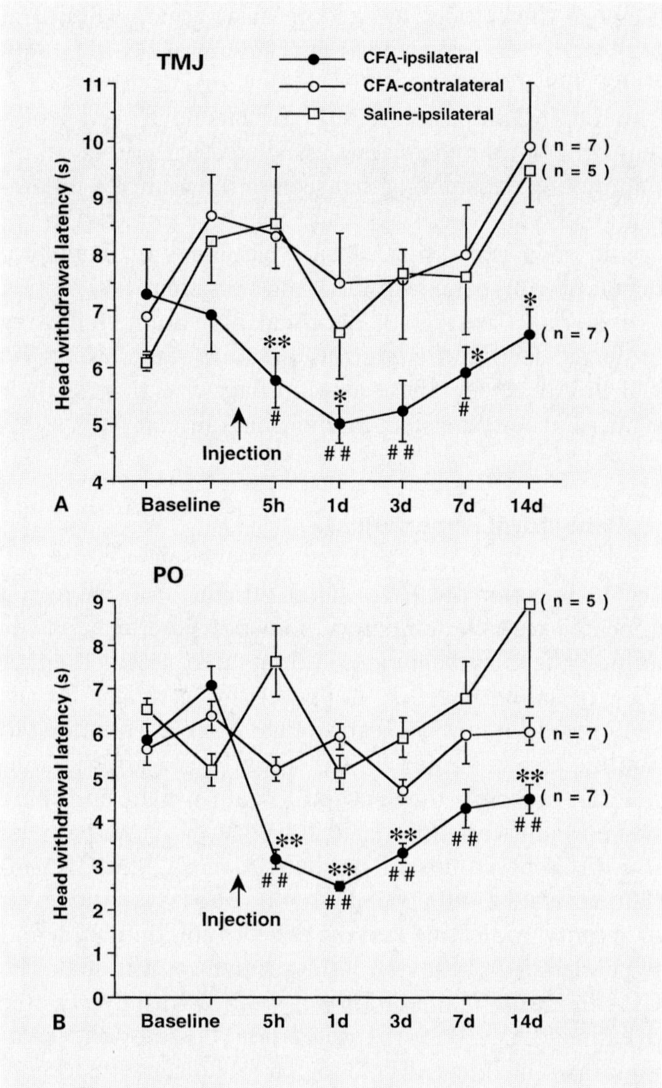

Fig. 1. Thermal hyperalgesia in CFA-inflamed rats. CFA (0.05 ml, 1:1 oil/saline suspension) was injected into the TMJ (**A**) and the perioral skin (PO) (**B**), respectively. Normal saline (0.05 ml) was injected in separate experiments in other rats as a control. The thermal stimulus was applied to the skin above the TMJ (**A**) and to the PO skin (**B**). The rats were lightly anesthetized with pentobarbital sodium (20 mg/kg i.p.) during the test. Asterisks indicate significant differences in head withdrawal latencies between ipsilateral and contralateral sides: * $p < 0.05$; ** $p < 0.01$. Pound signs indicate significant differences in head withdrawal latencies after inflammation as compared to the baseline withdrawal latencies: # $p < 0.05$; ## $p < 0.01$.

ing CFA injection (fig. 1B) (ANOVA, $F_{5,25} = 25.57$, $p < 0.001$). The thermal hyperalgesia began to appear at 5 h post injection of CFA and persisted over the two-week testing period, although the magnitude of hyperalgesia gradually attenuated (fig. 1). The injection of saline into the TMJ (n = 5) and PO (n = 5) regions did not produce significant changes in HWL to the heat stimulus (fig. 1).

A mechanical allodynia was also detected in the orofacial region following orofacial inflammation [Ren, 1999]. The development of allodynia followed a pattern similar to that after hindpaw inflammation. The mechanical threshold, as assessed by von Frey filaments [Ren, 1999], started to reduce at 2 h after inflammation. The allodynia peaked between 4 and 24 h and persisted for at least 2 weeks. Not only was the mechanical response threshold reduced after inflammation, but the response pattern was also altered. Rats tended to have stronger responses to the probing, indicated by attempting to remove the von Frey hair with the forepaw, exaggerated withdrawal movement, and frequent facial grooming. Such a response profile suggests the presence of mechanical allodynia characterized by a nocifensive response to a non-noxious stimulus.

Previous studies have mainly used models of transient pain in the orofacial region. Formalin injected into the upper lip produces two phases of intense rubbing of the face that last less than one hour [Clavelou et al., 1989; Raboisson et al., 1995]. Mechanical and thermal stimuli have been applied to the face to produce transient pain [Rosenfeld et al., 1978; Morris et al., 1982; Cahusac et al., 1990]. Algesic chemicals have been applied to the TMJ of cats to activate TMJ afferents to study responses of trigeminal nociceptive neurons with effects lasting about 30–60 s [Broton et al., 1988]. More recently, mustard oil has been injected into the periarticular temporomandibular tissue of anesthetized rats, resulting in reflex hyperexcitability of the jaw and neck muscles for up to 20–30 min [Haas et al., 1992; Yu et al., 1995]. Compared to these models, the injection of CFA into the TMJ and PO skin produces inflammatory hyperalgesia and allodynia that persist for hours and days. We have used this model to study long-term changes in the central nervous system associated with ongoing hyperalgesia.

Preprodynorphin mRNA Upregulation

At the spinal level, the change in opioid mRNA levels and their peptide products in response to tissue inflammation has been extensively studied [Iadarola et al., 1988b; Millan et al., 1988; Ruda et al., 1988; Noguchi et al., 1991, 1992]. Preprodynorphin (PPD) and preproenkephalin (PPE) opioid levels are affected by inflammatory agents, such as CFA [Iadarola et al., 1988b; Ruda et al., 1988; Nahin et al., 1989; Przewlocka et al., 1992], carrageenan [Noguchi et al., 1991, 1992], and formalin [Noguchi et al., 1989]. Such noxious stimuli greatly increase PPD-mRNA expression and dynorphin peptide levels in the spinal cord but have less effect on PPE-mRNA and it's peptide product [Iadarola et al., 1988b; Noguchi et al., 1992; Przewlocka et al., 1992; Tokunaga et al., 1992]. Prolonged nociceptive stimulation induces release of the opioid peptides as well as their biosynthesis in the spinal cord [Przewlocka et al., 1992]. A few studies have examined opioid gene expression in response to trigeminal deafferentation [Nishimori et al., 1988], formalin injection into the upper lip [Tokunaga et al., 1992], and electrical stimulation of trigeminal ganglion [Nishimori et al., 1989]. Kato et al. [1995] reported the appearance of dynorphin in the spinal trigeminal nucleus (Vsp) following experimental tooth movement.

We have compared the effects of deep TMJ and cutaneous PO skin inflammation on opioid gene expression at the trigeminal level [Imbe and Ren, 1999]. RNA blot analysis of the tissues including the spinal trigeminal complex demonstrated a single hybridization band at the appropriate position for rat PPD mRNA or PPE mRNA (fig. 2). Consistent with previous studies, the constitutive expression of PPD mRNA was very low. Densitometric analysis of the RNA blots (n = 4) revealed that the PPD mRNA level ipsilateral to TMJ inflammation was increased by 56.5 ± 14.7% (n = 4) when compared to the contralateral side and the Naive group ($p < 0.05$). The PO inflammation only produced a 27.5 ± 9.8% increase in PPD mRNA on the side ipsilateral to CFA injection. This increase did not reach statistical significance ($p > 0.05$). Compared to PPD mRNA, the constitutive expression of PPE mRNA was much higher. Neither TMJ nor PO inflammation produced a significant change in PPE mRNA levels in the trigeminal-spinal complex. Saline injection did not produce a significant effect on PPD and PPE mRNA expression.

The distribution pattern of PPD and PPE mRNA-positive neurons was further localized by in situ hybridization histochemistry. Neurons exhibiting up-regulation of PPD mRNA were mainly distributed in the medial portion of laminae I–II (Vc and C1–3), the dorsal portion of Vsp, and the paratrigeminal nucleus (Pa5), ipsilateral to TMJ inflammation. The mean number of PPD positive neurons in these regions was significantly higher than that on the contralateral side. A portion of the TMJ inflammation-induced PPD mRNA positive neurons in the Vsp and Pa5 projected to the parabrachial nucleus [Imbe and Ren, 2000], suggesting that the selective upregulation of PPD mRNA reflects an increased excitability in ascending trigeminal nociceptive pathways. The effect of PO inflammation on PPD mRNA expression was less dramatic. In the PO-CFA group, PPD mRNA-positive neurons were only found in the intermediate portion of the ipsilateral Vc.

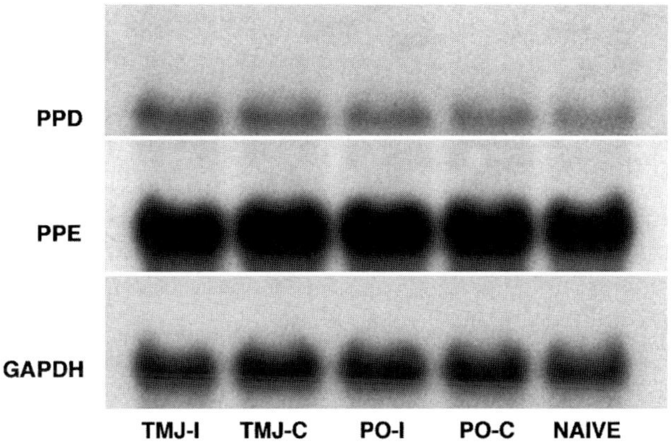

Fig. 2. Effects of TMJ and PO inflammation on PPD and PPE mRNA expression. RNA blots of PPD (upper), PPE (middle) and GAPDH (glyceraldehyde phosphate dehydrogenase, the lower bands, used as an RNA loading control) mRNAs are shown. Total RNA was extracted from a block of brain stem of the trigeminal spinal complex 2 mm rostral to 6 mm caudal to the obex. Adapted from Imbe and Ren [1999], with permission.

The TMJ is mainly innervated by branches of the auriculotemporal, masseteric, deep temporal, and lateral pterygoid nerves from the mandibular division of the trigeminal nerve [Klineberg, 1971]. When the location of the PPD mRNA-positive neurons in TMJ-CFA group was compared with previous HRP studies, it was found that the location of PPD mRNA-positive neurons was mainly within the region receiving mandibular projections, thus somatotopically relevant [Imbe and Ren, 2000]. This is consistent with previous results that the enhancement of PPD mRNA was in the area corresponding to the central somatotopic representation of the site of origin of the inflammation [Ruda et al., 1988; Noguchi et al., 1991; Tokunaga et al., 1992].

It is interesting that in TMJ-, but not PO-CFA inflamed rats, a significant number of PPD mRNA-positive neurons were identified in the ipsilateral Pa5. We also found that TMJ inflammation induced significant Fos protein expression in the ipsilateral Pa5 [Zhou et al., 1999]. The Pa5 is a large collection of interstitial neurons and neuropil in the spinal trigeminal tract at the level of the transition from the medullary dorsal horn to Vi [Phelan and Falls, 1989]. The Pa5 receives convergent sensory input from the head and neck as well as from the cranial portion of the alimentary tract [Armstrong and Hopkins, 1998]. The sensory inputs to the Pa5 are further relayed to other nuclei implicated in central pain pathways, such as the parabrachial nucleus [Bernard et al., 1989; Imbe and Ren, 2000]. The Pa5 also relays information from the peripheral area to the dorsal vagal complex [Armstrong and Hopkins, 1998]. Thus, Pa5 and neighboring Vi/Vc trigeminal transition may play an important role in the integration of deep sensory inputs with autonomic responses.

The upregulation of the PPD gene would enhance the activity of dynorphin-containing neurons and facilitate nociceptive transmission in the trigeminal pain pathways [Imbe and Ren, 1999; also see Ruda et al., 1995]. Compared to PO cutaneous inflammation, the injection of CFA into the TMJ resulted in greater upregulation of PPD mRNA expression. Consistently, TMJ inflammation induced significantly greater Fos protein expression than PO inflammation [Zhou et al., 1999].

Trigeminal Neuronal Hyperexcitability

We extended analysis of adjuvant-induced persistent orofacial inflammation to determine the long-term effects of such inflammation on subnucleus caudalis (Vc) neuronal activity [Iwata et al., 1999]. The Vc is the rostral extension of the upper cervical spinal dorsal horn and is also referred to as the medullary dorsal horn (MDH). Similar to the spinal dorsal horn, nociceptive specific (NS) neurons and some wide dynamic range (WDR) neurons are distributed in the superficial laminae, and most WDR neurons are found in the deep laminae of the MDH [Dubner and Bennett, 1983]. Nociceptive neurons excited by TMJ input are also classified as WDR and NS neurons and the receptive fields (RFs) of those neurons extend to wide areas of the facial skin and intraoral structures [Broton et al., 1988].

Medullary dorsal horn neurons were recorded extracellularly and classified as low-threshold mechanoreceptive, WDR and NS neurons according to their response properties to mechanical stimulation. To compare the effects of persistent deep joint and cutaneous orofacial injury, the inflammation was induced 24 h before the recordings by injection CFA into the TMJ capsule or the PO skin. The RFs of MDH nociceptive neurons were significantly enlarged after inflammation. The increases in RF size of WDR neurons after TMJ inflammation were greater than after PO inflammation. In TMJ-inflamed rats, the enlarged RFs were found both in neurons whose RFs included the facial skin over the TMJ as well as in neurons whose RFs were entirely outside the zone of injury. However, in PO-inflamed animals, the enlarged RFs always included the injured site and neurons with RFs located outside the injured region were not affected by CFA injection. This suggests a central convergence of deep and cutaneous nociceptors and referred excitation of cutaneous nociceptors after deep TMJ injury. Responses to thermal stimuli were significantly greater in inflamed animals than in naive animals in the 48–55 °C noxious range. Responses to nonnoxious and noxious mechanical stimuli were greater in inflamed as compared to naive rats and generally were greater after TMJ than PO inflammation. There was also an increase in background activity in MDH nociceptive neurons.

These results indicate that persistent orofacial inflammation produced hyperexcitability of MDH nociceptive neurons. TMJ inflammation resulted in greater changes in MDH nociceptive neurons as compared to PO inflammation, consistent with other findings of increased inflammation, increased MDH Fos protein expression, and increased MDH PPD mRNA expression in this orofacial model of inflammation and hyperalgesia [Imbe and Ren, 1999; Zhou et al., 1999]. At the spinal level, persistent input after inflammation leads to increased responsiveness to thermal and mechanical stimuli, an expansion of peripheral RFs, and an increase in background activity [Calvino et al., 1987; Shaible and Schmidt, 1988; Hylden et al., 1989; Woolf and King 1990; Ren et al., 1992]. The responses to longer lasting stimuli have been examined in trigeminal neurons [Hu et al., 1992; Yu et al., 1993; Raboisson et al., 1995; Meng et al., 1997; Iwata et al., 1999]. Following the application of mustard oil into the deep masseter, the RFs of MDH nociceptive neurons gradually expand and background activity is also significantly increased [Hu et al., 1992]. The findings from TMJ and PO inflammation model suggest a long-term trigeminal hyperexcitability that contributes to mechanisms of peristent pain associated with orofacial deep tissue painful conditions.

Fos Protein Expression

The stimulation-induced expression of Fos, the protein product of an immediate early gene, c-*fos*, has been widely used as a measure of nociceptive neuronal activation

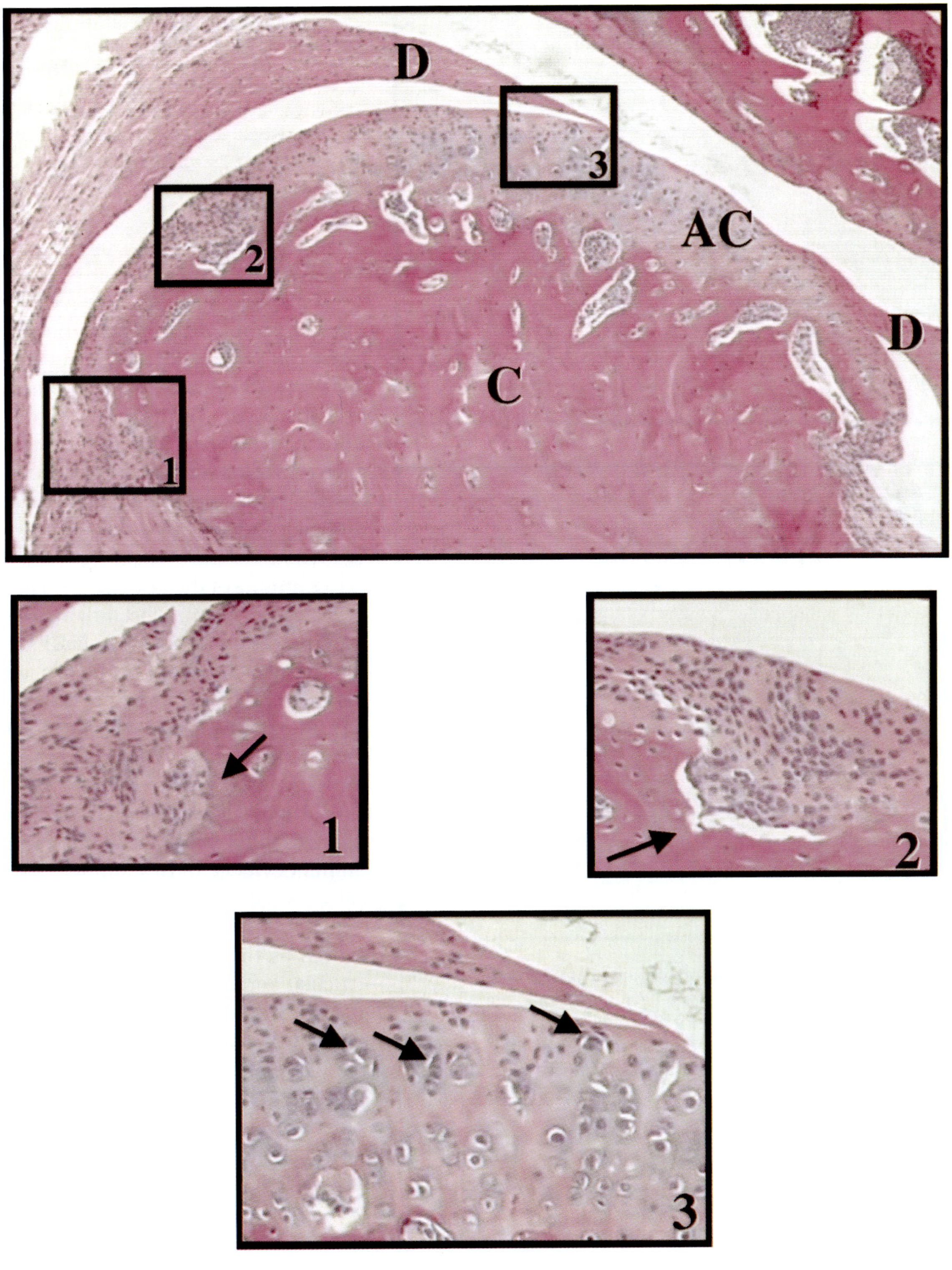

Fig. 1. Histological features of the transgenic mouse TMJ. The top panel is a low power HE view of the mouse TMJ. C = Condyle; D = disc; AC = articular cartilage. The numbered regions correspond to higher power view presented below. Regions of the joint undergoing bone resorption (panels 1 and 2, arrows) and proliferation and cloning of articular chondrocytes (panel 3, arrows) are evident.

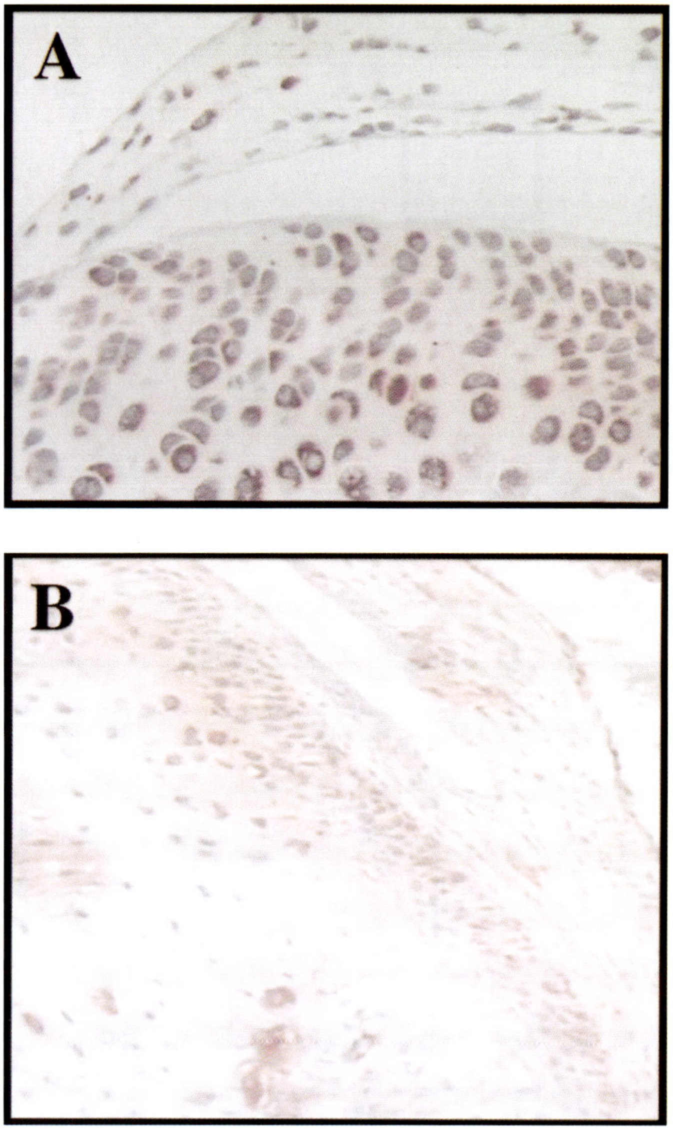

Fig. 2. Immunocytochemical localization of MMP9 and IL-1 in the transgenic mouse TMJ. **A** Articular chondrocytes and fibrochondrocytes of the disc expressing MMP9. The reddish-brown chromogen is localized in the cells and lacunae and is not present within the nuclei of the cells. **B** A more diffuse cellular and matrix staining for IL-1. Both the articular cartilage and disc are positive for this cytokine.

Histology

Formalin-fixed, decalcified, paraffin-embedded tissue from 8 transgenic and 8 control mice was obtained from 12-week-old animals. HE sections were reviewed for confirmation of an arthritic pathology. Immunohistochemical analysis was performed on 3-μm sections that were cut, deparaffinized and hydrated in graded alcohols. Endogenous peroxidase was blocked by immersion in 3% hydrogen peroxide for 10 min. Slides were rinsed in phosphate-buffered saline. Epitope enhancement was performed through microwave and/or trypsin digestion.

Sections were incubated overnight with primary antibodies in appropriate dilutions, and developed using a biotin-streptavidin protocol with AEC chromogen. Cytoplasmic deposition of chromogen was interpreted as positive immunostaining. Formalin-fixed sections of synovial tissue with active rheumatoid arthritis served as positive controls. Negative controls were prepared by omitting the primary antibody.

Results

Transgenic mice expressing a human TNF-α gene that has been altered to increase the stability of the TNF-α transcript show arthritic changes at a number of joints [4]. We have examined these animals to determine if the arthritis occurs in the TMJ as well. A histological and immunocytochemical analysis of the joint shows the presence of (i) clonal chondrocytes in the articular fibrocartilage; (ii) bone resorption around the periphery of the mandibular condyle; (iii) influx of inflammatory cells at the synovium; (iv) early fissuring of the condylar surface, and (v) a thinning of the disc (fig. 1). These are all features of a degenerating joint. The inflamed synovium is an early occurrence in the temporomandibular joint and precedes the structural changes in the articular fibrocartilage and disc. This type of synovium is a feature of rheumatoid arthritis, however, with further progression of the disease the changes resemble the advanced stages of osteoarthritis.

Virtually all articular cells and most of the fibrochondrocytes in the disc react with antibodies to MMP9. The immunocytochemical staining is localized to the individual cells with little appearing in the surrounding matrix (fig. 2A). A diffuse expression of IL-1 is present in the cells as well as the surrounding matrix. It appears that both articular and disc cells produce IL-1 (fig. 2B).

Conditioned medium from TMJ disc cells contains a number of enzymes with gelatinolytic activity. A gelatin zymogram from these cells demonstrates three marked activities, one at 92 kD, one at 72 kD, and one at 58 kD. These correspond to the 92K gelatinase (MMP9), the 72K gelatinase (MMP2) and one of the stromelysins, respectively. Other minor activities can be visualized on the zymogram and likely represent other MMPs. MMP9 in its zymogen form migrates as a 92-kD band (fig. 3A). Activation of this enzyme with the organo-mercurial, APMA, causes the enzyme to assume an open conformation and allows processing to a smaller 84-kD form (fig. 3B). A quantitative analysis of the two different forms of MMP9 indicates that APMA shifts that activity from the 92-kD form to the 84-kD form by at least fourfold and that chela-

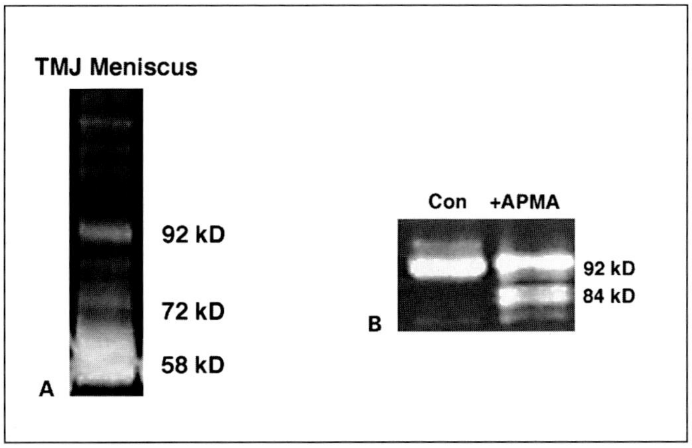

Fig. 3. Zymographic analyses of matrix metalloproteinase activity from TMJ disc cells. **A** The presence of three major gelatinolytic bands (92, 72 and 58 kD) and a number of lesser bands present in conditioned medium of TMJ disc cells. The band at 92 kD is MMP9. **B** Treatment of MMP9 with APMA, an organo-mercurial, will allow processing of the enzyme to the 84-kD form.

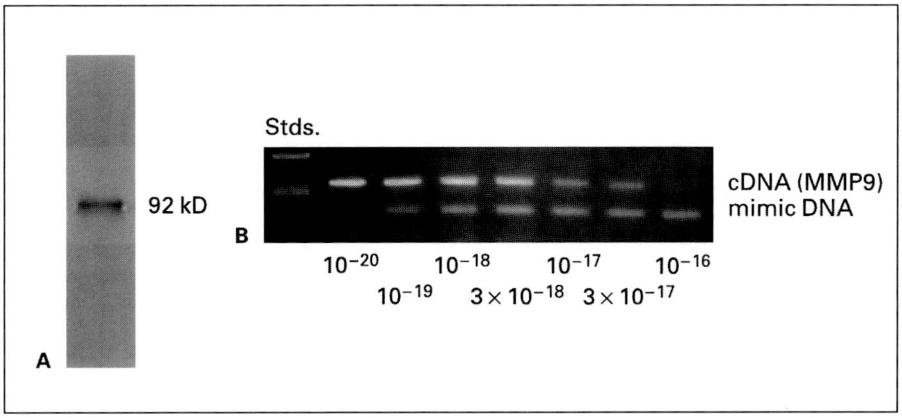

Fig. 4. Western immunoblot and RT-PCR identification of MMP9 from TMJ disc cells. **A** A single band identified by a specific polyclonal antibody (donated by William Stetler-Stevenson, NCI, NIH) at the expected molecular mass of 92 kD. **B** A quantitative PCR (qPCR) reaction identifying MMP9. Increasing amounts of a mimic DNA were amplified with the MMP9 cDNA using the same primer pair under identical conditions. Where the intensity of the mimic DNA and MMP9 cDNA bands are equal represents the amount of starting material for the MMP9 cDNA.

tion of calcium by EDTA and reduction of disulfide bonds by dithiothreitol eliminate any gelatinolytic activity at either 92 or 84 kD. All of these alterations in enzymatic activity are characteristic of MMP9 (fig. 3A).

Two other independent assays have both validated the presence of MMP9 in TMJ disc cells. Western blot analysis of conditioned medium from cells in culture demonstrate the presence of a single immunoreactive 92-kD band using an antibody specific for MMP9 (fig. 4A). Quantitative RT-PCR for the identification of MMP9 was performed (fig. 4B). A calculation of mRNA levels from this figure approximates the amount of mRNA to be 4.6×10^{-21} mol/cell or nearly 3,000 transcripts of MMP9 per cell. This calculation was performed by plotting the change in optical density for both the MMP9 cDNA and the MMP9 mimic as a function of the amount of mimic in the starting reaction. Where the two regression lines cross (i.e. where the MMP9 cDNA and MMP9 mimic DNA bands are of equal intensity), the starting amount of mimic cDNA equals the amount of MMP9 DNA in the sample. There are a number of variables however, that could influence the estimate of the number of transcripts per cell, such as RNA extraction efficiency, reverse transcriptase efficiency, and losses due to handling. All of these variables, however, would tend to decrease the amount of cDNA in the RT-PCR reaction tubes. Thus the estimate of 3,000 transcripts per cell, if in error, is likely to underestimate the amount.

The enzymatic activity of MMP9 in disc cells is regulated by TGF-β, IL-1 and prostaglandins (fig. 5). These data indicate that both TGF-β and IL-1 can stimulate MMP9 activity by over 10-fold in 24 h. PGE_2, on the other hand, is inhibitory for MMP9 activity. Statistically significant effects were seen with TGF-β and IL-1 in the low ng/ml range, a concentration that can occur in vivo. A greater than 90% inhibition of MMP9 activity by PGE_2 occurs at concentrations between 10^{-7} and 10^{-6} *M*. At this time we do not know if this effect is mediated at the transcriptional, translational or posttranslational level.

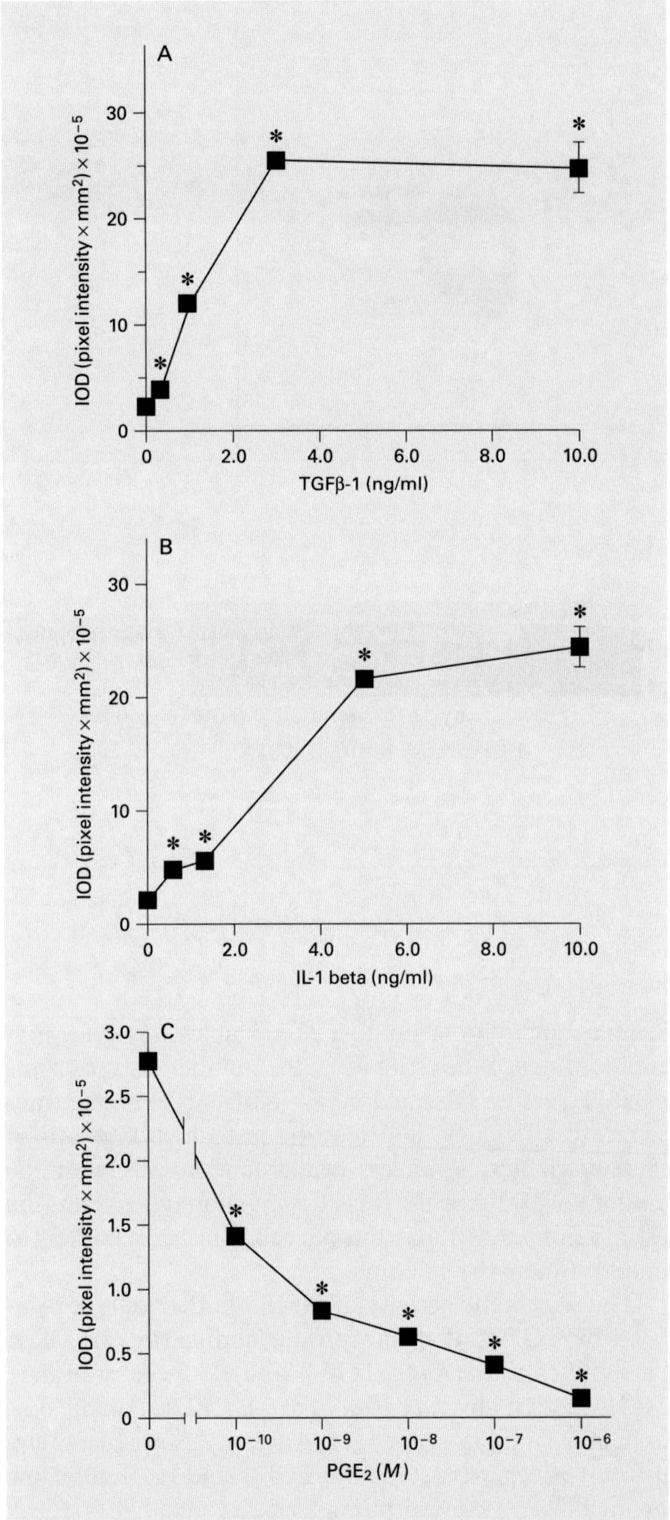

Fig. 5. Effect of cytokines on MMP activity. **A, B** TGF-β and IL-1 (10 ng/ml) stimulate MMP9 activity by over 10-fold after a 24-hour exposure. **C** PGE_2 inhibits MMP9 activity by over 90% between 10^{-6} and 10^{-7} *M*. Integrated optical density (IOD) was computed by multiplying the average pixel density for each MMP9 band times the number of pixels in the image. Each point represents the mean ± one SEM with n = 4. Where error bars are not evident, the SEM was smaller than the size of the point. * Statistically significant difference from control to treated cells to at least the $p \leq 0.05$ level.

Discussion

There is no good small animal model for TMJ arthritis. An animal surrogate in which there is a reproducible progression of degenerative joint disease would be of great value. However, such an animal, with pathology consistent with a purely osteoarthritic joint, seems beyond the scope of our technology at the present time. Thus, we have chosen to investigate the features of a transgenic mouse that acquires a polyarthritis within 6–12 weeks. The details of the construction of the transgene and genesis of this mouse have been described in the literature [5].

The early stages of arthritis in the knee and TMJ of this animal appear to be rheumatoid in nature. There is swelling of the joints accompanied by a synovial proliferation. However, within a few months, degradative characteristics of osteoarthritis appear. That is, articular chondrocytes begin to proliferate and form clonal colonies within the articular cartilage. Fissuring of the articular surfaces begins and thinning of the disc occurs. The progressive stages of arthritis in these mice do indeed resemble the advanced stages of osteoarthritis in the TMJ and knee.

Our immunocytochemical, biochemical and molecular data indicate that TMJ disc cells are capable of synthesizing MMP9 in a regulated fashion and that at least one of the cytokines involved in the regulation (i.e. IL-1) can be produced in the joint. Zymographic analysis of articular disc cell supernatants revealed the presence of at least three proteins (92, 72, 58 kD) with gelatinolytic activity. Traditionally, defining the enzyme characteristics of the MMPs with inhibitors and activators has assisted in their classification [17, 18]. Such an analysis has allowed us to document the likely identity of one of the proteins as MMP9. The fact that such activity is present may not be surprising since the presence of MMP enzymes in other types of articular tissues has been previously described. Mohtai et al. [18] studied human cartilage and documented the presence of the 92-kD as well as the presence of the 72-kD gelatinase with its two activated forms (66 and 62 kD).

resorption models [Seckinger et al., 1990]. Thus, increasing IL-1ra levels could potentially be helpful. The fact that TMD patients have significantly higher levels of IL-1ra suggests that the body is naturally trying to combat the inflammation and bony changes, but that the levels of IL-1ra produced are not sufficient to overcome the increased levels of IL-1β in the TMJ.

It has been reported that IL-10 can inhibit the production of several of the proinflammatory cytokines studied here including TNFα, IL-1, IL-6, and IL-8. Unfortunately, IL-10 levels were undetected in both control and TMD patients, suggesting that IL-10 production is not being upregulated in response to the increased levels of the proinflammatory cytokines [Fang et al., 1999]. Perhaps if it were clinically feasible to supplement or upregulate IL-10 it could help in the treatment of TMD.

Therefore, proinflammatory cytokine inhibitors such as TNF receptors, receptor antagonists (IL-1ra), and inhibitory cytokines (IL-10) may be important in controlling inflammation, connective tissue destruction, and bone loss in synovial joints like the TMD. Finally, it appears that to prevent/treat the pathological condition of TMD, a delicate balance must be reached/restored between proinflammatory cytokines and their inhibitors.

References

Alstergren, P., M. Ernberg, M. Kvarnstrom, S. Kopp (1998) Interleukin-1β in synovial fluid from the arthritic temporomandibular joint and its relation to pain, mobility, and anterior open bite. J Oral Maxillofac Surg *56:* 1059–1065.

Arend, W.P., J.M. Dayer (1990) Cytokines and cytokine inhibitors or antagonists in rheumatoid arthritis. Arthritis Rheum *33:* 305–315.

Dayer J-M. (1991) Chronic inflammatory joint diseases: Natural inhibitors of interleukin 1 and tumor necrosis factor α. J Rheumatol *18:* 71–75.

Dijkgraaf, L.C., L.G.M. de Bont, G. Boering, R.S.B. Lim (1995) Normal cartilage structure, biochemistry, and metabolism: a review of the literature. J Oral Maxillofac Surg *53:* 924–929.

Espevik, T., J. Nissen-Meyer (1986) A highly sensitive cell line, WEHI 164 clone 13, for measuring cytotoxic factor/tumor necrosis factor from human monocytes. J Immunol Methods *95:* 99–105.

Fang, P-K., X-C. Ma, D-L. Ma, K-Y. Fu (1999) Determination of interleukin-1 receptor antagonist, interleukin-10, and transforming growth factor-β1 in synovial fluid aspirates of patients with temporomandibular disorders. J Oral Maxillofac Surg *57:* 922–928.

Feldmann, M., F.M. Brennan, R.N. Maini (1996) Role of cytokines in rheumatoid arthritis. Annu Rev Immunol *14:* 397–440.

Firestein, G.S., D.L. Boyle, C. Yu, M.M. Paine, T.D. Whisenand, N.J. Zvaifler, W.P. Arend (1994) Synovial interleukin-1 receptor antagonist and interleukin-1 balance in rheumatoid arthritis. Arthritis Rheum *37:* 644–652.

Fort, J. (1999) Celecoxib, a COX-2-specific inhibitor: the clinical data. Am J Orthoped *28:* 13–18.

Fu, K., X. Ma, Z. Zhang, W. Chen (1995) Tumor necrosis factor in synovial fluid of patients with temporomandibular disorders. J Oral Maxillofac Surg *53:* 424–426.

Garrison, L., N.D. McDonnell (1999) Etanercept: Therapeutic use in patients with rheumatoid arthritis. Ann Rheumatic Diseases *58:* I65–69.

Guerne, P.A., B.L. Zuraw, J.H. Vaughan, D.A. Carson, M. Lotz (1989) Synovium as a source of interleukin 6 in vitro. J Clin Invest *83:* 585–592.

Haraldson, T., R. Jonsson, A. Tarkowski (1988) Spontaneous temporomandibular joint arthropathy in MRL-Ipr/Ipr mice. J Oral Pathol *17:* 386–389.

Holmlund, A., A. Ekblom, P. Hansson, J. Lind, T. Lundeberg, E. Theodorsson (1991) Concentration of neuropeptides substance P, neurokinin A, calcitonin gene-related peptide, neuropeptide Y and vasoactive intestinal polypeptide in synovial fluid of the human temporomandibular joint. Int J Oral Maxillofac Surg *20:* 228–231.

Holmlund, A.B., G. Gynther, F.P. Reinholt (1992) Rheumatoid arthritis and disk derangement of the temporomandibular joint. Oral Surg Oral Med Pathol *73:* 273–277.

Horai, R., S. Saijo, H. Tanioka, S. Nakae, K. Sudo, A. Okahara, T. Ikuse, M. Asano, Y. Iwakura (2000) Development of chronic inflammatory arthropathy resembling rheumatoid arthritis in interleukin 1 receptor antagonist-deficient mice. J Exp Med *191:* 313–320.

Koch, A.E., S.L. Kunkel, J.C. Burrows, H.L. Evanoff, G.K. Haines, R.M. Pope, R.M. Strieter (1991) Synovial tissue macrophage as a source of the chemotactic cytokine IL-8. J Immunol *147:* 3347–3353.

Kong, Y.Y., U. Feige, I. Sarosi, B. Bolon, A. Tafuri, S. Morony, C. Capparelli, J. Li, R. Elliott, S. McCabe, T. Wong, G. Campagnuolo, E. Moran, E.R. Bogoch, G. Van, L.T. Nguyen, P.S. Ohashi, D.L. Lacey, E. Fish, W.J. Boyle, J.M. Penninger (1999) Activated T cells regulate bone loss and joint destruction in adjuvant arthritis through osteoprotegerin ligand. Nature *402:* 304–309.

Kopps, S. (1998) The influence of neuropeptides, serotonin, and interleukin 1β on temporomandibular joint pain and inflammation. J Oral Maxillofac Surg *56:* 189–191.

Kubota, E., H. Imamura, T. Kubota, T. Shibata, K. Murakami (1997) Interleukin 1β and stromelysin (MMP3) activity of synovial fluid as possible markers of osteoarthritis in the temporomandibular joint. J Oral Maxillofac Surg *55:* 20–27.

Kubota, E., T. Kubota, J. Matsumoto, T. Shibata, K.I. Murakami (1998) Synovial fluid cytokines and proteinases as markers of temporomandibular joint disease. J Oral Maxillofac Surg *56:* 192–198.

Lennard, A.C. (1995) Interleukin-1 receptor antagonist. Crit Rev Immunol *15:* 77–105.

Moore, K.W., A. O'Garra, R. de Waal Malefyt, P. Vieira, T.R. Mosmann (1993) Interleukin-10. Annu Rev Immunol *11:* 165–190.

Nicod, L.P., P. Isler, R. Chicheportiche, F. Songeon, J.M. Dayer (1996) Production of prostaglandin E2 and collagenase is inhibited by the recombinant soluble tumor necrosis factor receptor p55-human gamma 3 fusion protein at concentrations a hundred-fold lower than those decreasing T cell activation. Eur Cytokine Netw *7:* 757–763.

Sandler, N.A., M.J. Buckley, J.E. Cillo, T.W. Braun (1998) Correlation of inflammatory cytokines with arthroscopic findings in patients with temporomandibular joint internal derangements. J Oral Maxillofac Surg *56:* 534–543.

Seckinger, P., S. Isaaz, J-M. Dayer (1998) A human inhibitor of tumor necrosis factor α. J Exp Med *167:* 1511–1516.

Seckinger, P., S. Isaaz, J-M. Dayer (1989) Purification and biologic characterization of a specific tumor necrosis factor α inhibitor. J Biol Chem *264:* 11966–11973.

Seckinger, P., J. Klein-Nulend, C. Alander, R.C. Thompson, J-M. Dayer, L.G. Raisz (1990) Natural and recombinant human IL-1 receptor antagonists block the effects of IL-1 on bone resorption and prostaglandin production. J Immunol *145:* 4181–4184.

Shafer, D.M., L. Assael, L.B. White, E.F. Rossomando (1994) Tumor necrosis factor-α as a biochemical marker of pain and outcome in temporomandibular joints with internal derangements. J Oral Maxillofac Surg *52:* 786–791.

Stegenga, B., L.G.M. de Bont, G. Boering (1989) Osteoarthritis as the cause of craniomandibular pain and dysfunction: A unifying concept. J Oral Maxillofac Surg *47:* 249–256.

Takahashi, T., T. Kondoh, M. Fukuda, Y. Yamazaki, T. Toyosaki, R. Suzuki (1998) Proinflammatory cytokines detectable in synovial fluids from patients with temporomandibular disorders. Oral Surg Oral Med Oral Pathol Oral Radiol Endod *85:* 135–141.

van Leeuwen, M.A., J. Westra, P.C. Limburg, P.L.C.M. van Riel, M.H. van Rijswijk (1995) Interleukin-6 in relation to other proinflammatory cytokines, chemotactic activity and neutrophil activation in rheumatoid synovial fluid. Ann Rheum Dis *54:* 33–38.

Van Zee, K.J., T. Kohno, E. Fischer, C.S. Rock, L.L. Moldawer, S.F. Lowry (1992) Tumor necrosis factor soluble receptors circulate during experimental and clinical inflammation and can protect against excessive tumor necrosis factor α in vitro and in vivo. Proc Natl Acad Sci. USA *89:* 4845–4849.

Walmsley, M., P.D. Katsikis, E. Abney, S. Perry, R.O. Williams, R.N. Maini, M. Feldmann (1996) Interleukin-10 inhibition of the progression of established collagen-induced arthritis. Arthritis Rheum *39:* 495–503.

Cells
Tissues
Organs

Cells Tissues Organs 2001;169:265–271

Drug Discovery and Target Validation

Mark E. Nuttall

Department of Bone and Cartilage Biology, GlaxoSmithKline Pharmaceuticals, King of Prussia, Pa., USA

Key Words
Drug discovery · Pharmaceuticals · Genomics · Proteomics

Abstract
Recent drug discovery has been driven largely by a genomics-based approach. This revolution in pharmaceutics is based on localized expression of either a novel gene or homologue of a known gene found in cDNA libraries made from normal versus diseased tissue. The choice and quality of cDNA library is critical for the success of this approach. Expression is normally verified at the cellular level by either immunocytochemistry or in situ hybridization. Activity of the recombinant protein in secondary cell-based assays allows highthroughput screens to be formulated to identify small-molecule effectors of this protein. More recently, a proteomics approach has also been incorporated into this process. This technology directly measures proteins whose expression is localized in disease tissue as the basis for cell-based screens to look for either activators or inhibitors, of this activity. The majority of screens are designed to look for inhibitors. Activity of small-molecules found by screening gives rise to pharmacokinetic studies and verification of activity in animal models of the disease. Structure-activity relationship (SAR) optimization of these small-molecules allows for suitable oral bioavailability and pharmacokinetics, resulting in compounds progressing from discovery to development. Based on these strategies, we have developed inhibitors of osteoclast-mediated bone resorption and are currently screening for bone anabolic agents. In addition, we have also developed small-molecule caspase inhibitors which prevent chondrocyte apoptosis and retain cell function in an attempt to find therapeutic agents to either prevent or treat osteoarthritis. These agents may well have utility in the treatment of temporomandibular joint diseases.

The Drug Discovery Process

The process of drug discovery and validation has been revolutionized by the evolving role of genomics-based target discovery. This has occurred as a result of recent advances in high throughput genomic sequencing which has allowed large-scale analysis of the profile of expressed genes in a given cell type. This process enables the sequencing of low-abundant genes from specialized cell types (i.e. osteoclasts, neuronal cells) and thus a direct comparison between normal versus diseased tissues or

KARGER
Fax + 41 61 306 12 34
E-Mail karger@karger.ch
www.karger.com

1422–6405/01/1693–0265$17.50/0

Accessible online at:
www.karger.com/journals/cto

Mark E. Nuttall, PhD
GlaxoSmithKline Pharmaceuticals, UW2109
709 Swedeland Road, King of Prussia, PA 19406 (USA)
Tel. +1 610 270 4998, Fax +1 610 270 5598
E-Mail mark_e_nuttall@sbphrd.com

control versus drug-treated cells. Because of the ability to amplify genomic material, the number of cells required for an adequate analysis of expressed genes in a particular cell type is small. One of the major factors in this approach is the choice and quality of cDNA library. Contaminating cells can confuse the analysis of genes found expressed in a library. One way to overcome this is to make a secondary library consisting entirely of mRNA from cells from the contaminating component of the original mixture. The whole process of target discovery and validation is extensive and involved. Therefore, the preparation of high-quality human cDNA libraries from homogeneous cell populations results in the discovery of genes that can ultimately provide successful disease targets.

Alternatives to mass sequencing of cDNA's is comparative analysis of expression using techniques such as DNA microarrays, transcript imaging, differential display, representative difference analysis (RDA) and serial analysis of gene expression (SAGE) [El-Meanawy et al., 2000; Rogge et al., 2000; Tollett-Egnell et al., 2000; Wang et al., 2000]. It is beyond the scope of this report to compare the relative merits of each gene discovery technique, but suffice to say that they all have their advantages and pitfalls and are suited to particular projects depending on availability and quality of the starting biological material.

A brief overview of the idealized process is shown in figure 1 and a conservative estimate from gene discovery to 'drug in human' is 10 years. It must be emphasized that this simplified overview of the drug discovery process is for the idealized identification of small-molecule orally active compounds against classic targets (i.e. receptors, enzymes) and this does not in any way capture the variations in this path nor the peculiar hurdles that each target presents.

Once the novel gene or homologue is identified, expression is usually confirmed by either northern blot or polymerase chain reaction (PCR) analysis of the RNA in the cell or tissue of interest. This is then confirmed more specifically in terms of individual cell expression of mRNA by in situ hybridization or protein by immunocytochemistry (if there is an antibody available). These are both powerful techniques that confirm expression in mixed-cell populations on tissue sections. Once expression has been confirmed, the gene is usually expressed in an artificial expression system such as baculovirus, yeast, bacteria *(Escherichia coli)* or mammalian cells (i.e. Chinese hamster ovary, HeLa). The protein is purified from this expression system and a screen established. The screen is based on the nature of the target. For example, a membrane receptor screen may be simply binding to the receptor or modulation of downstream signaling from this receptor, whereas for a protease it could be based on inhibition of peptide cleavage in an artificial system where the protease is recombinantly expressed. Screens are high-throughput (robotic-based in 96-, 384- or 1,536-well microtitre plates) on compound collection banks (usually >100,000 compounds), although depending on the nature of the target, 'biased' or subsets of screening banks can be examined more thoroughly. Recent advances in combinatorial chemistry has allowed many compounds to be synthesized rapidly and these are usually screened as mixtures of derivatives from an original molecular template [Gordon et al., 1994]. Hits from mixtures are de-convoluted to allow identification of the particular compound within that set which is a hit. Hits from this chemically diverse compound collection are then tested in secondary assays which are usually in vitro assays preferably using a cell expressing the endogenous protein. The readout from these secondary assays is often a 'biological endpoint' such as proliferation, differentiation or apoptosis. The potency of these hits can be increased by chemical modification therefore enhancing the structure-activity relationship (SAR). These are then either tested directly in animal models, if suitable disease models are available, or drug metabolism and pharmacokinetic studies (DMPK) are performed to test cell permeability and oral availability. Suitable DMPK profiles then allow animal testing and proof-of-concept in animal studies. This is a crucial tier of selection because of solubility, instability and cell-permeability issues associated with small-molecules in biological fluids and their ability to transverse cell membranes. Success at this stage allows toxicology profiles and safety medicine studies, and, if these prove positive in terms of safety to man then the drug is ready to be tested in humans.

The drug discovery process is considerably more complicated than that presented in a simple flow diagram (fig. 1). In figure 2, we have tried to capture some of the synergies that must occur during this process. Possibly, the major supporting technology for target validation is genetic manipulation, where knockout/overexpression or directed expression of a particular gene may provide very powerful evidence to support a role for that gene product in a particular disease. As this technology develops and the regulated switching 'on and off' of genes can occur in the already developed animal, the results will be even stronger evidence for a role for specific targets in disease states.

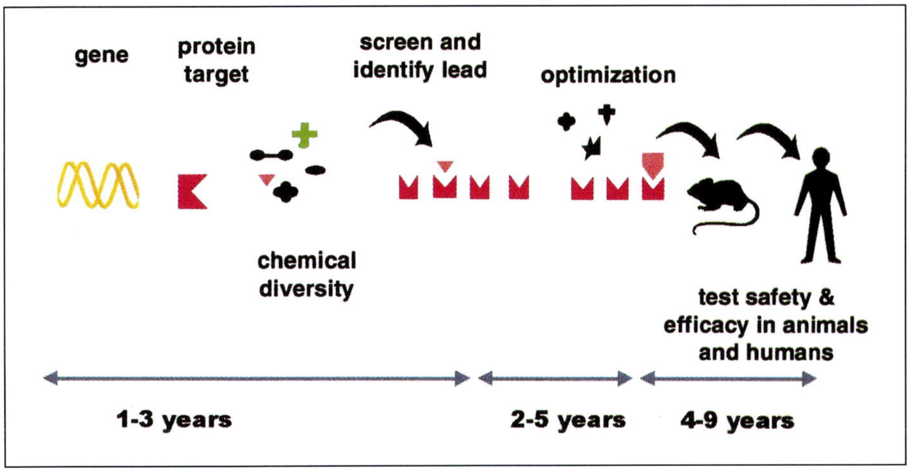

Fig. 1. The drug discovery process.

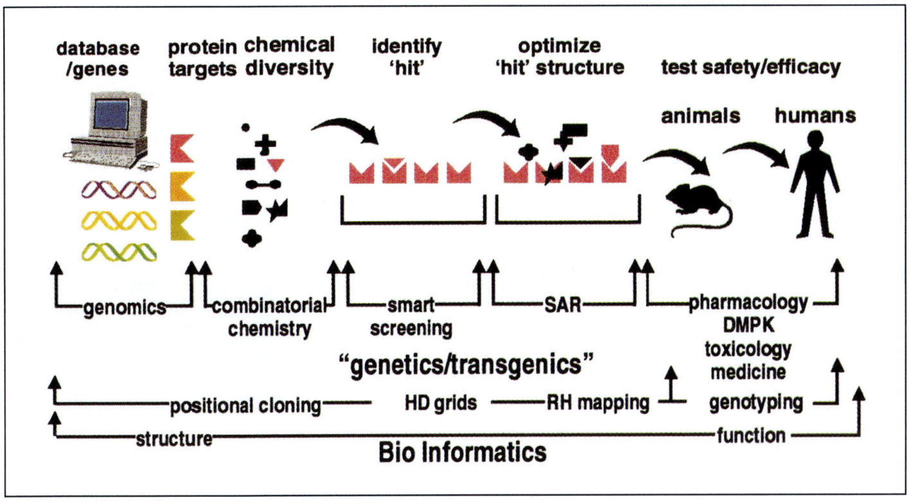

Fig. 2. Key steps in the drug discovery process.

As well as transgenics, there is now considerable investment in bioinformatics not only for gene discovery, but also for continued gene surveillance and database monitoring during the target validation process. As we near the completion of sequencing of the genome, the power of bioinformatics increases, especially when comparing genomes of different species which allows extensive homologue searching across species.

Drug Discovery Efforts Based on Restricted Expression

A successful example on this type of approach was the discovery of the novel cysteine protease cathepsin K from a human osteoclast cDNA library [Drake et al., 1996]. This protease comprised approximately 4% of the sequences found in this library after extensive cDNA sequencing (>5,000 expressed sequence tags). Immunocytochemistry and in situ hybridization confirmed the localized and high expression of this gene in osteoclasts from human osteoclastoma (fig. 3a). There was high expression only in bone, osteoclastoma, resorbing cartilage and synovium from osteoarthritic patients. A drug discovery effort can be validated based on exclusive expression of a gene in a particular cell type that can be associated with a disease process of sufficient commercial interest. The working model for cathepsin K is that this protease is secreted into the lumen at the osteoclast bone interface where it degrades the bone matrix (fig. 3b). This therefore provides a target to inhibit bone resorption and thus prevent the bone loss that occurs during osteoporosis. These data have culminated in a full discovery effort by a number of pharmaceutical and biotechnology companies.

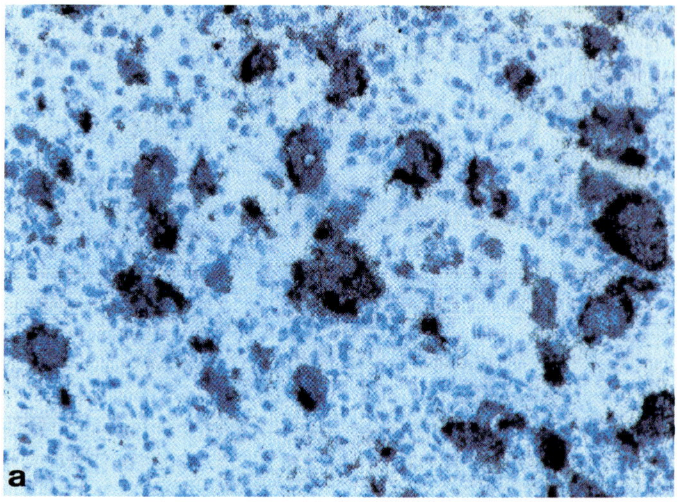

Fig. 3. **a** Human osteoclastoma in situ hybridization for cathepsin K [Drake et al., 1996]. **b** Model to indicate the release of cathepsin K at the osteoclast bone interface where matrix degradation takes place.

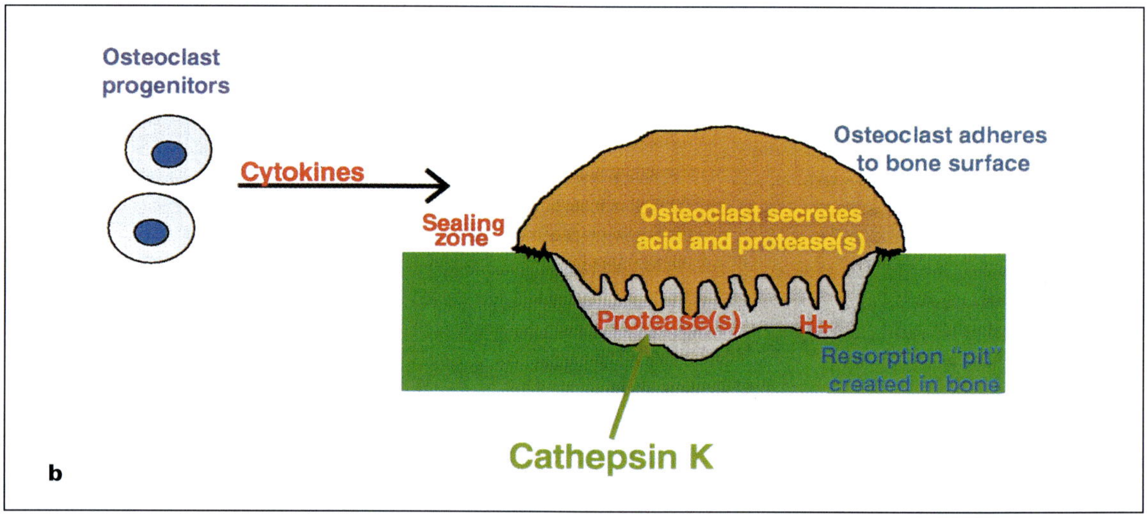

Drug Discovery Based on Homology Searching

Several novel homologues of the Ced-3 gene were found in cDNA databases. Ced-3 is a *Candida elegans* gene which when knocked out was shown to prevent cell death in the developing nematode [Ellis and Horvitz, 1986]. The tissue distribution of these homologues gave no indication as to restricted expression and therefore their involvement in particular disease processes was unknown. However, their criticality in the apoptotic process had been proven in the nematode gene knockout studies [Ellis and Horvitz, 1986]. We therefore established smart screens for inhibitors and discovered small-molecule inhibitors of the cysteine protease caspase 3. These were then tested in disease models in which there was evidence of dysregulated apoptosis. One of these compounds (compound A; fig. 4), which was based on SAR studies around the structure of a hit from the screen, which originally had low micromolar potency, was found to inhibit chondrocyte apoptosis. Compound A was found to be a specific inhibitor of caspases 3 and 7 and inhibited caspase 3 and 7 with Ki_{app}'s of 15 and 47 nM, respectively [Lee et al., 2000]. This isatin sulfonamide exhibited 100-fold greater selectivity for the highly homologous caspases 3 and 7 versus all other family members except caspase 9 (10- to 50-fold). Based on its potency and selectivity, this compound provides unique opportunity to determine the relevance of caspases 3 and 7 in diseases known to be associated with dysregulated apoptosis. Compound B is a structural analogue with considerably less potency at inhibiting caspases (Ki_{app}'s of 12 μM against caspase 3).

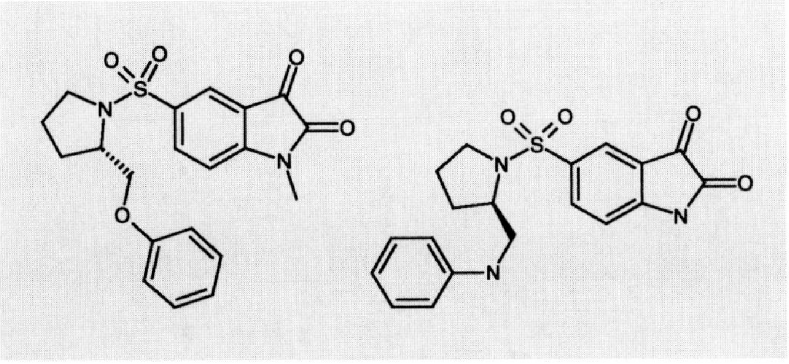

Fig. 4. Caspase inhibitors.

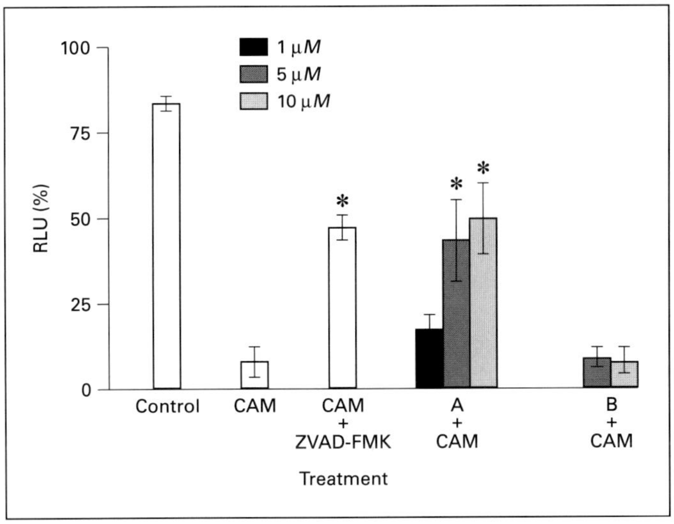

Fig. 5. Maintenance of type II collagen promoter activity after apoptotic insult in the presence of a caspase inhibitor. Primary bovine chondrocytes transiently transfected with a construct in which the regulatory sequences (–577 to +3,426) of the type II collagen (COL2A1) gene are driving luciferase reporter gene expression [Nuttall et al., 2000]. Cells were grown in serum-containing medium as a control (control). Cells were treated with 4 μg/ml of the apoptotic agent camptothecin (CAM) or 4 μg/ml CAM plus varying concentrations of compound A or B for 24 h. ZVAD-FMK is a nonselective caspase inhibitor. Expression of the COL2A1 gene was measured by luciferase activity measurements using a luminometer. Results are expressed as relative light units (RLU). Results are mean ± SD (n = 3). * $p < 0.02$, compared to CAM treatment alone.

The inhibition of chondrocyte apoptosis was significant because these cells, the only cell type found in cartilage, have been shown to undergo increased apoptosis in animal models of OA and increased apoptosis has been measured in clinical samples from osteoarthritic patients [Kouri et al., 1997; Blanco et al., 1998; Hashimoto et al., 1998]. OA is a chronic degenerative disease characterized by erosion of matrix and a reduction in chondrocyte cell number [Mankin et al., 1971]. Significantly, as well as inhibiting the death of these cells, the activity of the type II collagen promoter, the major extracellular matrix component of cartilage, was maintained (fig. 5). This suggests that as well as apoptosis being inhibited, the cells are still able to make matrix and therefore are functionally intact. This has important implications for the use of inhibitors of this activity in prevention of this disease process in the sense that the cells that remain are functional and are not 'ghost cells' with dysregulated gene expression profiles.

Therefore, based on the evidence of dysregulated apoptosis in OA and the evidence that caspases 3/7 inhibitors block chondrocyte cell death and retain matrix production of these cells, we believe that the inhibition of caspase activity provides a genome initiated novel therapeutic approach to either prevent or treat OA.

Proteomics Approach to Drug Discovery

The proteome is the protein content of a cell, tissue or entire organism in a defined state. Proteomics is the global analysis of protein expression using strategies that detect and quantitate changes in protein expression levels (fig. 6). Similar to genome analysis, this gives a 'snap-shot' of proteins present at any one time [Pandey and Mann, 2000]. The advantages of this approach are that events in cellular recognition and signal transduction occur at the protein level (e.g. antigen recognition, cell adhesion, and receptor binding). Although the majority of gene regulation in eukaryotes is at the level of transcriptional control, this is not exclusively so and translational control and protein stability effect activities of these genes. Functional proteomics allows the identification of protein interacting partners and can therefore identify multi-protein complexes. It is clearly emerging that multi-protein complexes (e.g. nuclear hormone receptors) play key roles in gene regulation.

There are technical challenges to the proteomics approach such as solubility of proteins, detection of only highly expressed proteins, no amplification system for proteins (viz. PCR for cDNA) and differential effects of post-translational modification on a protein's gel migration. Also the throughput and automation is as yet not comparable to genomic approaches.

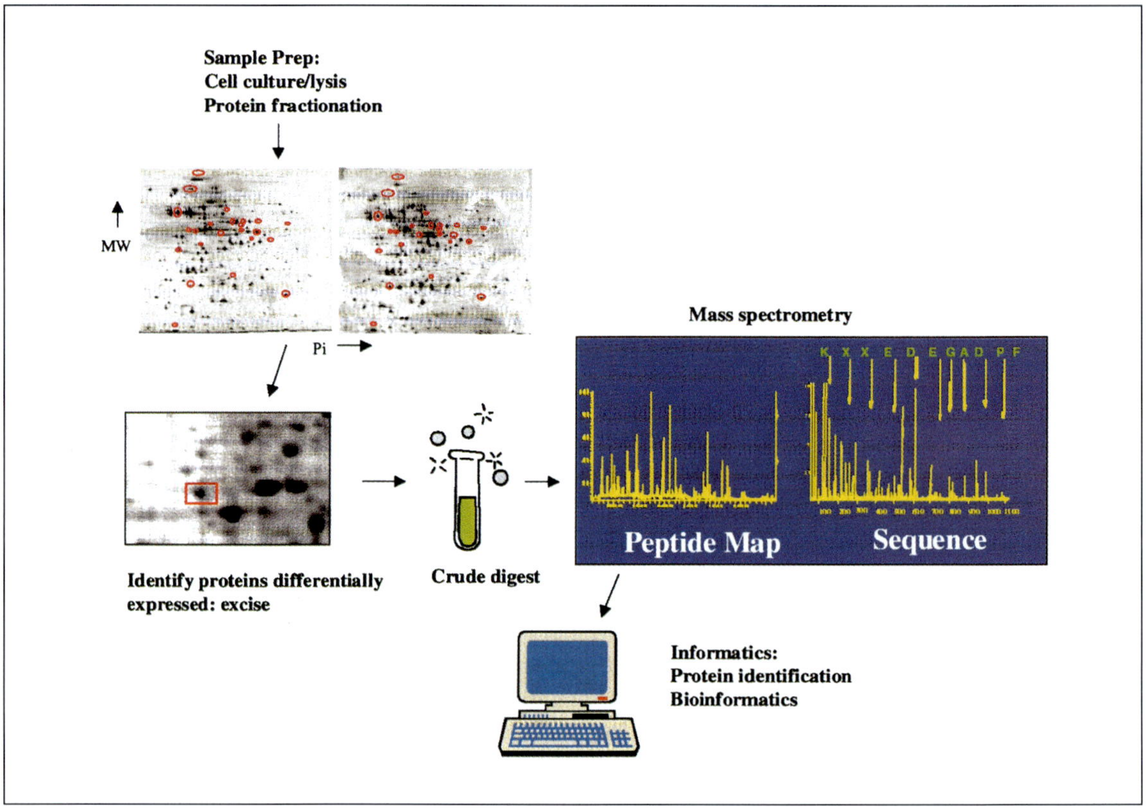

Fig. 6. The proteomics process.

However as sequencing of the genome is completed, a new approach will be to develop catalogs of protein interactions within a given cell, tissue or organism [Lander, 1996].

Clearly, proteomics approaches will play a crucial role in understanding protein-protein interactions.

How Could These Approaches Be Applicable for Identification of a Biological Target for TMJ?

Isolation of tissues (muscle and/or bone) from joints of patients with TMJ would allow mRNA isolation and cDNA preparation that could be used directly for cDNA library generation and mass sequencing. Alternatively, comparative techniques could be used, such as differential display or RDA, which have been used successfully on small amounts of tissue to identify genes that are regulated in diseases compared to normal tissue [Wang et al., 2000]. With the currently available new library amplification procedures very little tissue is needed (<1 μg total RNA). It seems unlikely that there would be enough material at this stage for a proteomics approach. However, as technology improves, it may be possible in the future to miniaturize and automate this process.

The two examples provided above, the cathepsin K and caspase 3/7 inhibitors are potential novel therapeutics to either prevent or treat TMJ. The development of these compounds would depend on certain biological observations. For the cathepsin K inhibitor, excessive bone resorption with cathepsin K expression would need to be shown in this disease compared to tissue from non-diseased individuals to warrant moving forward with this kind of antiresorptive strategy. For the caspase 3/7 inhibitors, excessive apoptosis would, at the very least, need to be shown in the tissues of TMJ patients. This increased cell death could occur from damage to either the muscle or bone in the affected joints. The next step would be to show a caspase 3/7-dependent mechanism of action in this tissue.

The potential of compounds currently on the market for skeletal diseases, i.e. bisphosphonates, selective estrogen receptor modulators, and compounds in development, i.e. cathepsin K and anti-apoptotic compounds may well have potential for the treatment of TMJ. However, before these can be tested clinically a thorough understanding of this disease process is required. This may be achievable by harnessing the new technologies and drug discovery processes described in this report.

In summary, the availability of genomic (and in future proteomic) techniques will allow identification of novel molecular targets from relatively small amounts of tissue. In diseases such as TMJ where tissue is limiting, these may prove very powerful approaches to discover novel therapeutic targets to either prevent or treat this disease.

Acknowledgements

I would like to thank Dr. Larry Suva for critical reading of the manuscript. I would also like to thank Janice Connor and Dr. R.A. Dodds for use of their cathepsin K in situ hybridization plate.

References

Blanco, F.J., R.L. Ochs, H. Schwarz, M. Lotz (1995) Chondrocyte apoptosis induced by nitric oxide. Am J Pathol *146:* 75–85.

Drake, F.H., R.A. Dodds, I.E. James, J.R. Connor, C. Debouck, S. Richardson, E. Lee-Rykaczewski, L. Coleman, D. Rieman, R. Barthlow, G. Hastings, M. Gowen (1996) Cathepsin K, but not cathepsins B, L, or S, is abundantly expressed in human osteoclasts. J Biol Chem *271:* 12511–12516.

Ellis, H.M., H.R. Horvitz (1986) Genetic control of programmed cell death in the nematode *C. elegans*. Cell *44:* 817–829.

El-Meanawy, M.A., J.R. Schelling, F. Pozuelo, M.M. Churpek, E.K. Ficker, S. Iyengar, J.R. Sedor (2000) Use of serial analysis of gene expression to generate kidney expression libraries. Am J Physiol *279:* 383–392.

Gordon, E.M., R.W. Barrett, W.J. Dower, S.P.A. Fodor, M.A. Gallop (1994) Applications of combinatorial technologies to drug discovery: Combinatorial organic synthesis, library screening strategies and future directions. J Med Chem *37:* 1385–1401.

Hashimoto, S., R.L. Ochs, S. Komiya, M. Lotz (1998) Linkage of chondrocyte apoptosis and cartilage degradation in human osteoarthritis. Arthritis Rheum *41:* 1632–1638.

Kouri, J.B., J.L. Rosales-Encina, P.P. Chaudhuri, J. Luna, R. Mena (1997) Apoptosis in human osteoarthritic cartilage: A microscopy report. Med Sci Res *25:* 245–248.

Lander, E.S. (1996) The new genomics: Global views of biology. Science *274:* 536–539.

Lee, D., S.A. Long, J.L. Adams, G. Chan, K.S. Vaidya, T.A. Francis, K. Kikly, J.D. Winkler, C.-M. Sung, C. Debouck, S. Richardson, M.A. Levy, W.E. De Wolf, Jr., P.M. Keller, T. Tomaszek, M.S. Head, M.D. Ryan, R.C. Haltiwanger, P.-H. Liang, C.A. Janson, P.J. McDevitt, K. Johanson, N.O. Concha, W. Chan, S.S. Abdel-Meguid, A.M. Badger, M.W. Lark, D.P. Nadeau, L.J. Suva, M. Gowen, M.E. Nuttall (2000) Potent and selective nonpeptide inhibitors of caspases 3 and 7 inhibit apoptosis and maintain cell functionality. J Biol Chem *270:* 16007–16014.

Mankin, H., H. Dorfman, L. Lippiello, A. Zarins (1971) Biochemical and metabolic abnormalities in articular cartilage from osteoarthritic human hips: Correlation of morphology and metabolic data. J Bone Joint Surg *53:* 523–537.

Nuttall, M.E., D.P. Nadeau, P.W. Fisher, F. Wang, P.M. Keller, W.E. De Wolf, M.B. Goldring, D. Lee, M.A. Levy, M. Gowen, M.W. Lark (2000) Inhibition of caspase-3-like activity prevents apoptosis while retaining functionality of human chondrocytes in vitro. J Orthop Res *18:* 356–363.

Pandey, A., M. Mann (2000) Proteomics to study genes and genomes. Nature *405:* 837–846.

Rogge L., E. Bianchi, M. Biffi, E. Bono, S.Y.P. Chang, H. Alexander, C. Santini, G. Ferrari, L. Sinigaglia, M. Seiler, M. Neeb, J. Mous, F. Sinigaglia, U. Certa (2000) Transcript imaging of the development of human T helper cells using oligonucleotide arrays. Nat Genet *25:* 96–101.

Tollet-Egnell, P., A. Flores-Morales, J. Odeberg, J. Lundeberg, G. Norstedt (2000) Differential cloning of growth hormone-regulated hepatic transcripts in the aged rat. Endocrinology *141:* 910–921.

Wang, F.-L., J.C. Connor, R.A. Dodds, I.E. James, S. Kumar, M.W. Lark, M. Gowen, M.E. Nuttall (2000) Differential expression of Egr-1 in osteoarthritic compared to normal adult human articular cartilage. Osteoarthritis Cartilage *8:* 161–169.

Cells Tissues Organs

Cells Tissues Organs 2001;169:272–278

Photopolymerized Biomaterials for Application in the Temporomandibular Joint

Amy K. Poshusta[a] Kristi S. Anseth[a,b]

[a]Department of Chemical Engineering, and [b]Howard Hughes Medical Institute, University of Colorado, Boulder, Colo., USA

Key Words

Biomaterials · Photopolymerization · Tissue engineering · 3-D prototyping · Temporomandibular joint

Abstract

Chronic foreign body reactions have limited the successful application of alloplastic implants for treatment of temporomandibular joint (TMJ) disorders. There is a great clinical need for new materials with enhanced properties for application in the diarthrodial joint. Photopolymerizations may provide many advantages for fabricating new biomaterials for the TMJ and may address some of the notable differences between the TMJ and other articulations. Specifically, the feasibility of trans-tissue (i.e. through the skin) photopolymerizations may yield less-invasive surgical procedures. Also, novel 3-dimensional photoprocessing techniques may be used to fabricate patient-specific alloplastic devices for improved compliance and efficacy. Finally, the mild conditions necessary for photopolymerizations make the reaction ideal for encapsulating cells with the potential to create constructs for tissue engineering, which may be beneficial for disk replacement therapies.

Introduction

Diseases and deformities of the temporomandibular joint (TMJ) may result in a variety of symptoms ranging from pain, myalgia, headache, bone resorption, hypomobility, occlusional changes, and joint displacement. Surgical treatment for symptomatic relief may include reconstruction of the fossa, condyle, condyloid process, or ramus of the mandible, and most often involves removal of the joint's meniscus. However, following meniscectomy, complications (e.g. degenerative joint disease, fibrous ankylosis and pain) may result if a material is not interdisposed between the head of the condyle and the glenoid fossa. A majority of alloplastic meniscal implants were fabricated in the 1980s from Silastic (Dow Corning, Inc.) or Teflon-Proplast (Vitek, Inc.). However, these implant materials were shown to fragment under functional conditions [Kent et al., 1993; Wolford, 1997] producing wear

Abbreviations used in this paper

TMJ	temporomandibular joint
3-D	three-dimensional
LCD	liquid crystal display

K.S. Anseth, PhD
Howard Hughes Medical Institute
University of Colorado
Boulder, CO 80309-0424 (USA)
Tel. +1 303 492 3147, Fax +1 303 492 4341, E-Mail kristi.anseth@colorado.edu

Cells
Tissues
Organs

Cells Tissues Organs 2001;169:279–284

Bone Blood Flow and Vascular Reactivity

John T. Fleming Michelle T. Barati Dennis J. Beck James C. Dodds
Arthur L. Malkani Dushi Parameswaran Galia K. Soukhova Michael J. Voor
Jeremy B.A. Feitelson

Osteohemodynamics Lab, Department of Physiology and Biophysics, and Department of Orthopaedic Surgery,
University of Louisville, Louisville, Ky., USA

Key Words
Bone · Blood flow · Endothelin · Norepinephrine · Injury

Abstract
Blood flow is essential for normal bone growth and bone repair. Like other organs, the regulation of blood flow to bone is complex and involves numerous physiologic mechanisms including the sympathetic nervous system, circulating hormones, and local metabolic factors. Our studies addressed the following questions: (1) Which endogenous vasoconstrictor agents regulate in vivo blood flow to bone? (2) Does a decrease in bone vascular reactivity to vasoconstrictor hormones account for the increase in blood flow during bone healing? (3) Does the endothelium influence bone arteriolar function? An intact bone model was developed in the rat to assess hormonal regulation of in vivo bone blood flow and in vivo bone vascular reactivity. An isolated, perfused bone arteriole preparation was employed to characterize the responsiveness of small resistance-size arterioles (diameter $< 100\ \mu m$) to vasoconstrictor hormones and to evaluate the role of the vascular endothelium to modulate vascular smooth muscle reactivity. Our results indicate that: (1) though exogenous endothelin is a potent constrictor of the in vivo bone vasculature, endogenous endothelin does not actively regulate in vivo blood flow; (2) the increase in blood flow to a bone injury site is not due to a decrease in bone vascular sensitivity to norepinephrine, and (3) isolated bone arterioles of young rats are very sensitive to vasoconstrictor hormones but exhibit only modest endothelium-mediated vasodilation.

Abbreviations used in this paper

ET-1	endothelin-1
PU	perfusion units

Introduction

Clinical and laboratory research has clearly established a vascular linkage between bone metabolism, bone mechanics, and bone pathology [Brookes and Revelle, 1998]. According to Brinker et al. [1990]: 'Normal growth, remodeling, and repair of bone require delivery of nutrients and oxygen through blood flow to bone.' Therefore, inadequate blood flow to skeletal structures, including the temporomandibular joint, could impair normal development and/or healing processes.

KARGER
Fax +41 61 306 12 34
E-Mail karger@karger.ch
www.karger.com

Accessible online at:
www.karger.com/journals/cto

John T. Fleming, PhD
Department of Physiology and Biophysics
School of Medicine, University of Louisville
Louisville, KY 40292 (USA)
Tel. +1 502 852 5374, Fax +1 502 852 6239, E-Mail John.Fleming@Louisville.edu

Like other organs, the regulation of bone blood flow (osteohemodynamics) is complex and involves numerous physiologic mechanisms including the sympathetic nervous system, circulating hormones, and local metabolic factors [Winet, 1996; Brookes and Revelle, 1998]. Others have clearly demonstrated that exogenous norepinephrine [Stein et al. 1958; Ye et al., 1993] and endothelin [Coessens et al. 1996; Briggs et al., 1998] constrict the bone vasculature, confirming the presence of functional alpha-adrenergic and endothelin receptors. However, the design of their studies does not provide any indication of the extent to which endogenous norepinephrine or endothelin constricts vessels that supply blood to bone in vivo. Our studies have attempted to identify the endogenous vasoconstrictor hormones that regulate in vivo blood flow to bone. Our approach was to measure changes in bone blood flow after the administration of pharmacological agents that selectively inhibit alpha-adrenergic receptors or endothelin receptors. The extent to which in vivo blood flow increases after receptor blockade reflects the degree to which endogenous norepinephrine or endothelin is exerting a tonic constriction of the bone resistance vessels. Using this approach, we observed that inhibition of alpha-adrenergic receptors with phentolamine or phenoxybenzamine results in a significant decrease in bone vascular resistance (unpublished data), suggesting that endogenous norepinephrine controls basal blood flow via a tonic constrictor effect on the bone vasculature. In this article, we present findings regarding the role of endogenous endothelin to regulate in vivo blood flow to bone.

Blood flow also plays a vital role in the repair of bone following injury. According to Rhinelander [1974]: 'the two most essential factors in bone healing are stabilization of the osseous fragments and blood flow'. After a bone fracture, blood flow to the injury site changes to meet the metabolic needs of the healing tissue. Within the first few days, blood flow to the fracture site decreases substantially. But by 2 weeks later, blood flow increases substantially and remains elevated for several weeks [Laurnen and Kelly, 1969]. This sustained increase in flow is essential for normal bone union [Trueta, 1974], and is partially the result of angiogenesis within the fracture area [Glowacki, 1998]. However, we hypothesized that pre-existing vessels, adjacent to the fracture site, also play a role to increase flow to the site of repair. We investigated the possibility that vessels adjacent to the injury site become less sensitive to normal constrictor influences and therefore become partially relaxed, permitting an increase flow to the injury site. Since endogenous norepinephrine appears to exert a tonic constrictor effect on the bone vasculature, we proposed that the arterioles adjacent to the injury might become less responsive to the constrictor effects of norepinephrine. Thus, we compared the sensitivity of the bone vasculature to norepinephrine adjacent to the injury site and at a proximal diaphyseal site of healthy bone on the same femur.

In addition to the in vivo assessments of bone vasculature function, an isolated, perfused arteriole preparation was developed to evaluate the constrictor and dilator reactivity of bone arterioles (diameter < 100 μm), which regulate bone vascular resistance. This in vitro arteriole preparation allows for the control of intraluminal pressure, bath pH and temperature, bath concentrations of pharmacological agents, and for precise measurements of arteriole diameters in response to the topical application of vasoactive substances. Preliminary experiments were performed to determine: (1) if these arterioles were responsive to norepinephrine and endothelin, and (2) if the endothelium of these arterioles modulates vascular tone.

Materials and Methods

Hormonal Regulation of in vivo Bone Blood Flow

All animal protocols were approved by the Animal Care and Use Committee of the University of Louisville. Male Sprague-Dawley rats (wt. 340–410 g) from Harlan Inc. (Indianapolis, Ind., USA) were housed in the AALAC-approved Animal Care facility of the University of Louisville. The rats had access to food and water ad libitum. On the day of the experiment, each rat was anesthetized with Inactin (100 mg/kg i.p.). The left carotid artery was cannulated to measure arterial blood pressure. A cannula was inserted into the right iliac artery and advanced to the bifurcation of the aorta. The right iliac artery was occluded distal to the cannula so that drugs injected via the cannula would be delivered directly into the left hind limb circulation. The left tibia was exposed at a midshaft position by surgical incision. Approximately 5 mm of soft tissue and periosteum were removed to expose the cortex. A laser Doppler flow probe, connected to an Advance Laser (model ALF21R) Doppler flowmeter, was used to assess bone blood flow, a technique proven to be effective in measuring acute changes in bone perfusion [Lausten et al., 1993]. The probe was positioned against the exposed bone cortex and held in place by a micromanipulator. The preparation was allowed to equilibrate for one hour following the surgery. At critical phases of each experiment, a bone vascular resistance index (mm Hg/PU) was calculated by dividing the mean arterial blood pressure (mm Hg) by the laser Doppler perfusion units (PU).

First, a dose-response curve to ET-1 was generated by injecting five doses (0.05–10 μg) into the left hind limb vasculature while quantitating changes in arterial blood pressure and in vivo blood flow to the tibia. Second, an endothelin-A receptor antagonist (BQ-123; 3.7 μg) or an endothelin-B receptor antagonist (BQ-788; 3.9 μg) was administered prior to injection of ET-1 (5 μg) to determine if this dose of receptor antagonist would significantly diminish the vascular response to exogenous ET-1. The dose of antagonist which blocks the actions of a relatively high dose of exogenous ET-1 should inhibit the actions of the lower endogenous levels of endothelin. In a third set of experiments, either BQ-123 (3.7 μg) or BQ-788 (3.9 μg) was injected alone among rats that had not been exposed to exogenous ET-1 to determine if receptor blockade altered basal blood flow to the bone.

Vascular Reactivity during Bone Repair

Male Sprague-Dawley rats were anesthetized with Ketaset/Acepromazine. Under aseptic conditions, a 1.8-mm circular, uni-cortical defect was created in the lateral distal diaphysis of the left femur to simulate a fracture. Three weeks later, the rats (wt. 360–450 g) were anesthetized and in vivo blood flow experiments were performed. A laser Doppler flow probe was positioned adjacent to the injury site or at a proximal site of healthy femur cortex. Following the measurement of basal bone blood flow and arterial pressure, seven doses of norepinephrine (0.0016–1.6 μg/kg) were administered into the left hindlimb to generate a dose-response curve to norepinephrine at the injury site and at the healthy bone site.

Bone Arteriole in vitro Experiments

Bone arterioles were removed from the femoral canal of male Sprague-Dawley rats using a stereomicroscope and transferred to a bath chamber filled with a MOPS-buffered physiologic solution at room temperature. Each arteriole was cannulated at both ends with glass micropipettes and secured with suture. The arteriole was perfused with the MOPS-buffered solution at 40 mm Hg while gradually warming the bath chamber to 37 °C. The image of the bone arteriole was displayed on a calibrated television screen using a closed-circuit television microscopy system and recorded on videotape for later analysis. After establishing the baseline diameter of the arteriole, known concentrations of norepinephrine or ET-1 were added to the bath. Maximal arteriole constrictor responses were measured to each dose of agonist.

In other experiments, the dilator responses of the arterioles to acetylcholine, an endothelium-dependent dilator, and to sodium nitroprusside, an endothelium-independent dilator, were compared. First, the arterioles were pre-constricted with phenylephrine, and then exposed to a maximally dilating concentration of acetylcholine (10^{-4} *M* bath concentration). After the dilator response was measured, the bath was washed several times with drug-free physiologic solution to remove phenylephrine and acetylcholine and allow the arterioles to return to control diameters. The same arterioles were again pre-constricted with phenylephrine, and then exposed to sodium nitroprusside (10^{-4} *M* bath concentration).

Results

In vivo Bone Blood Flow Regulation

The two highest ET-1 doses (5 and 10 μg) had significant, dose-dependent effects on blood pressure and bone blood flow. After injecting the 5-μg dose, mean arterial blood pressure decreased initially (15–25%) then increased above the baseline value (17–25%) for a prolonged period (more than 10 min). Likewise, bone vascular resistance (arterial blood pressure/bone blood flow) decreased initially, then significantly increased in response to ET-1. ET-1 (5 μg) increased resistance by 40 ± 9% (fig. 1), while 10 μg of ET-1 increased resistance by 382 ± 115%. Inhibition of ET-A receptors with BQ-123 significantly attenuated the increase in bone vascular resistance caused by ET-1 (fig. 1). After blockade of ET-B receptors with BQ-788, the initial decrease in bone vascular resistance caused by ET-1 was abolished, but the ensuing increase in resistance was unaffected. When the ET-A antagonist was administered alone to a separate group of rats that had not been exposed to exogenous ET-1, neither mean arterial blood pressure, basal bone blood flow nor bone vascular resistance significantly changed (fig. 2). Similarly, inhibition of ET-B receptors failed to change basal bone vascular resistance.

Vascular Reactivity at Site of Bone Injury

Three weeks after surgery, the margin of the circular injury on the femur diaphysis was visible, however, the wound was nearly healed. In every animal, the basal blood flow adjacent to the injury (2.37 ± 0.8 PU) was significantly higher than the flow measured at the healthy diaphyseal site on the same bone (0.88 ± 0.10 PU). Correspondingly, the basal vascular resistance at the injury site (84.4 ± 21.1 units) was significantly lower than at the healthy site (151.1 ± 19.5 units). This flow differential suggests that the healing process was still underway and that blood flow regulation was altered (increased) to the injury area. The bolus injection of norepinephrine caused dose-dependent increases in bone vascular resistance at the injury site and the healthy site (fig. 3). However, the dose-response curves to norepinephrine were not statistically different between the two sites.

In vitro Bone Arteriole Experiments

Responsiveness to Constrictor Agonists. Control bone arteriole diameters ranged from 60 to 130 μm, with an average of 95 ± 7.7 μm. The application of norepinephrine to the bath caused a dose-dependent constriction (fig. 4), with the highest concentration (10 μ*M*) reducing arteriole diameters by 58 ± 3.3%. After washing norepinephrine from the bath, the arterioles returned to previous baseline diameters. Endothelin-1 (1 n*M*) constricted the arterioles by 69 ± 4.8% (fig. 4), 1/10,000th the concentration required by norepinephrine to produce a similar degree of constriction.

Role of the Vascular Endothelium. In separate experiments, pretreatment with phenylephrine reduced the bone arteriole diameters from 83 ± 9 to 52 ± 5 μm. The maximal diameter after exposure to acetylcholine was 55 ± 5 μm, only a 5 ± 4% increase. After several bath washes, the arterioles returned to their previous basal

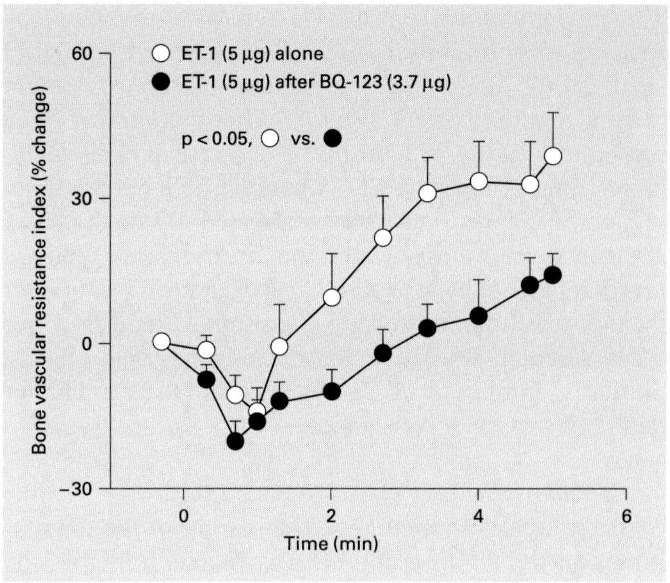

Fig. 1. Percent changes in the vascular resistance index (arterial pressure/laser Doppler perfusion units) of the intact rat tibia following injection of endothelin-1 alone (5 μg; n = 5) or to endothelin-1 (5 μg) after pretreatment with the endothelin-A antagonist, BQ-123 (3.7 μg; n = 5). The plotted values represent mean ± SEM values. The two dose-response curves were statistically different (ANOVA, $p < 0.05$).

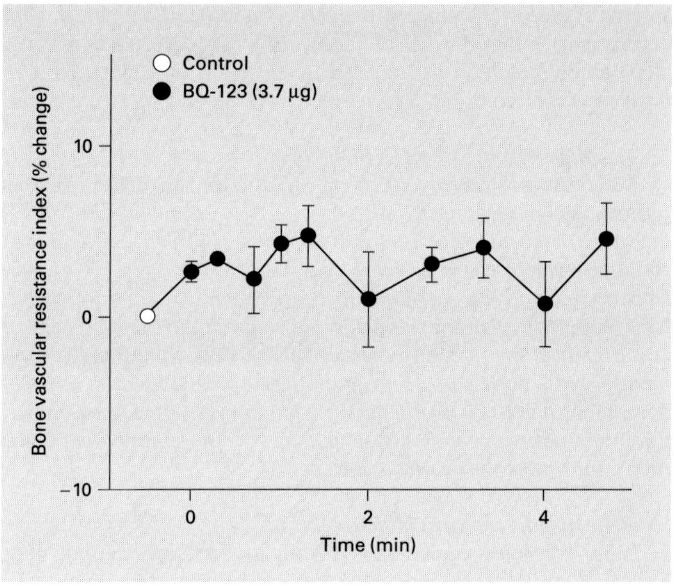

Fig. 2. The effect of BQ-123 (endothelin-A receptor antagonist) on the bone vascular resistance index of the intact rat tibia. The plotted values represent percent changes (mean ± SEM) from the control value (0%) obtained from 5 experiments. The resistance values after BQ-123 treatment were not statistically different from the basal resistance value. ANOVA, $p > 0.05$.

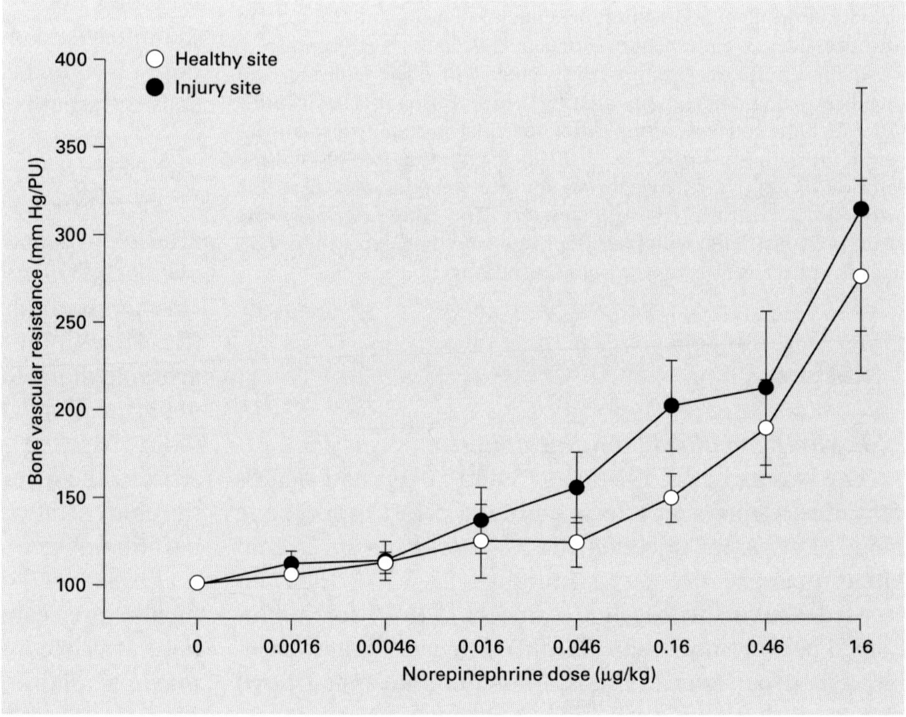

Fig. 3. Norepinephrine-induced increases in bone vascular resistance measured near the cortical injury or at a proximal site of healthy diaphysis on the same rat femur. The resistance changes at the two sites were not statistically different at any norepinephrine dose. The values represent mean ± SEM values obtained from five experiments.

implicated in the mediation of osteoclastogenesis [Bertolini et al., 1986; Gowen et al., 1990; Kimble et al., 1997]. Monocytic levels of TNF production have been shown to be elevated in surgical or natural menopausal states, and a number of studies have shown that TNF-α can induce osteoclast formation in vitro [Kimble et al., 1997]. More recently, both a novel member of the TNF receptor family, osteoprotegerin (OPG), and its specific ligand OPGL have been shown to be key regulators controlling bone mass through their regulation of the resorptive cycle [Simonet et al. 1997; Bucay et al., 1998; Lacey et al., 1998; Takahashi et al., 1999; Hofbauer et al., 2000]. Recent studies clearly indicate that apoptosis of chondrocytes plays an important role in endochondral ossification [Hashimoto et al., 1997; Horton et al., 1998]. Two members of the TNF family of cytokines, Fas ligand and TNF-α, have both been implicated in providing death signals to chondrocytes. Treatment of human articular chondrocytes with Fas ligand in vitro causes apoptosis and the Fas system has been shown to be present in growth plate chondrocytes in vivo, leading to the suggestion that it might play a role in chondrocyte apoptosis during endochondral development [Roach et al., 1996; Gibson et al., 1997; Lee et al., 1998]. In recent studies, our laboratories have shown that TNF-α can induce apoptosis in vitro in populations of growth chondrocytes [Aizawa et al., 2001]. A growing body of data has also shown that TNF-α plays a major role in the pathogenesis and destruction of joints in rheumatoid arthritis, suggesting that it has profound biological effects on normal cartilage metabolism [Lipsky et al., 2000]. The focus of the current studies was to determine the role of TNF-α in the mediation of either endochondral bone repair or intramembranous bone repair.

Materials and Methods

Materials

Histological reagents and chemicals were purchased either from Sigma Chemical Company (St Louis, Mo., USA) or Fisher Scientific (Springfield, N.J., USA). RPA reagents were from PharMingen Corp. (San Diego, Calif., USA). Homozygous knock-out mice in which the genes for both TNF-α receptors ($p55^{-/-}/p75^{-/-}$) were targeted [Peschon et al., 1998] and strain matched controls were from Jackson Laboratories (Bar Harbour, Me., USA). C3H10T½ mesenchymal stem cells were obtained from American Type Culture Collection (Rockville, Md., USA). Pathogen-free eggs were purchased from Spafas Farms (Storrs, Conn., USA). All tissue culture supplies were from either Sigma or Gibco BRL Life Technologies (Grand Island, N.Y., USA). Transwell Culture Devices were from Millipore Corp (Medford, Mass., USA).

Production of Simple Transverse Fractures and Marrow Ablation

Eight- to ten-week-old male knock-out mice and matched control mice were used for this study. Closed, transverse, mid-diaphyseal fractures of the tibiae were generated by controlled blunt trauma using a modification of the technique developed for rats [Bonnarens and Einhorn, 1984; Hiltunen et al., 1993]. The tibia was chosen for used in the mouse versus the femur in the rat, since for this species it provides better anatomic features than the femur for the performance of the fracture procedure [Hiltunen et al., 1993]. Fracture stabilization by intramedullary fixation was carried out using the trochar of a 25-G and 23-G spinal needle.

Tibia marrow ablation was performed as described by Suva et al. [1993]. Briefly, mice were anesthetized by inhalation with isoflurane. A small incision along the medial aspect of the proximal muscle overlying the tibia was made and the muscle retracted to expose the bone. A small 1-mm hole was drilled through the cortex into the marrow space. A 23-G needle was then inserted the length of the marrow cavity and gently rotated to disrupt the marrow cavity. The marrow contents were removed by vacuum suction and the space flushed with sterile saline. Following ablation the site was closed with suture. The animals were permitted full weight-bearing and unrestricted activity after awakening from anesthesia for both models of bone repair. Mice were euthanized by cervical dislocation on various days over a 28-day period as reported in the results.

Histology

At the time of euthanasia, the fracture sites or marrow ablated bones were recovered and fixed for 3 days in 4% para-formaldehyde in phosphate-buffered saline at 4°C. Specimens were completely decalcified in Immunocal (Decal Chemical Corporation, Congers, N.Y., USA) and embedded in paraffin. The tissue was appropriately positioned in paraffin to make sagittal sections and cut at 6 μm thickness. Sections were stained with hematoxylin and eosin.

Preparation of Avian Skeletal Cell Populations

Chondrocyte populations enriched in hypertrophic and non-hypertrophic cells were prepared from sternae of 17-day-old chick embryos and cultures were grown as previously described [Gerstenfeld et al., 1989]. Co-cultures were initiated with second passage chick embryo cephalic sterna chondrocytes.

Co-Culture with C3H10T½

C3H10T½ cells were plated at 2.5×10^4 cells per 33-mm diameter culture wells and maintained in DMEM 10% FBS for 24 h. At the end of this second 24-hour period, the medium was removed and the cultures were replenished with fresh medium. Co-culture was carried out using Millipore trans-well devices with 45 μm size exclusion. Co-cultures were initiated 48 h after plating by placing the trans wells, pre-seeded with 2.5×10^5 avian effector cells, into the wells of the 33-mm dishes overlying the responder C3H10T½ cells. All measurements were made after 21 days of growth under co-culture conditions. All cell cultures were maintained in DMEM, 10% FBS unless otherwise noted.

RNA Analysis

RNA was isolated from cells or from knock-out and control animals. Animal tissues were collected in duplicate sets of pooled samples [n = 10 (days 1 and 3) and n = 5 (days 7, 14, 21 and 28)]. Bones were retrieved on the indicated days after fracture or marrow ablation and powdered under liquid nitrogen with a mortar and pestle.

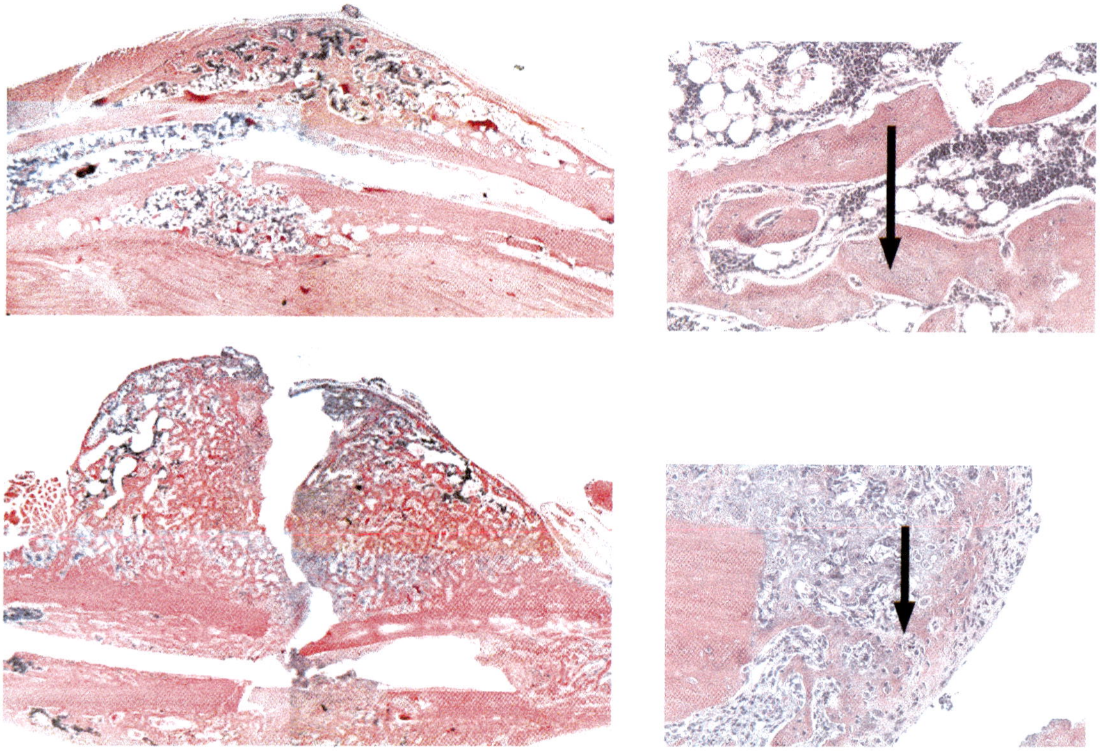

Fig. 1. Selected histological analysis of fracture repair of wild-type and TNF-α receptor TNFR $p55^{-/-}/p75^{-/-}$ deficient mice. Days after fracture are indicated in the figure. **A** Low 50 × magnification of the panoramic view of the fracture repair at day 21 after fracture. Note the dramatic differences in size of the calluses at 21 days. **B** Higher 200 × magnification of 21 days at the fracture site highlighting the failure to induce periosteal induced membranous bone repair. The site of fracture is denoted with an arrow.

The total RNA was extracted from the powdered tissues or cells with Tri-Reagent™ (Molecular Research Center Inc., Cincinnati, Ohio, USA) as previously described [Toma et al., 1997]. RNA quantities were determined by $OD_{260\,nm}$ and sample integrity was monitored by visualization of ribosomal RNAs with ethidium bromide after denaturing RNA gel electrophoresis [Thomas, 1980].

RNase Protection Analysis

Messenger RNA expression during fracture healing was quantitatively assessed by ribonuclease protection analysis (RPA). Linearized plasmids for mouse collagen types I, II and X, osteocalcin, L32 and GAPDH were purchased from PharMingen Corp. (San Diego, Calif., USA). Single stranded ^{32}P-labeled cRNA probes were generated using RNA transcription kits purchased from PharMingen Corp. as per the manufacturer's instructions. RNase protection products were fractionated on a denaturing 6% acrylamide gel [Gerstenfeld et al., 1989]. The autoradiographic bands of the RNase protection products were quantified using an Alpha Innotech Image Analysis System, Alpha Innotech, Inc. Underexposed autoradiographic images were used for all analyses and the autoradiographic densities of the protected bands from each probe were measured. The quantities of individual mRNAs for specific cytokines and extracellular matrix proteins were determined in the following manner. It was assumed that each probe had the same specific activity (i.e., the same ratio of radiolabeled nucleotides are incorporated for each run-off product) and that the annealing efficiencies between all the probes and their target mRNA sequences were the same under the conditions used in these studies. All data were normalized to either a so-called housekeeping gene such as glyceraldehyde-3-phosphate dehydrogenase (GAPDH) or L32 mRNA.

Results

The role of TNF-α in endochondral bone formation was first assessed by comparing fracture repair in normal and knock-out mice deficient in both p55/p75 TNF-α receptors. Dramatically altered fracture healing was observed in the TNF $p55^{-/-}/p75^{-/-}$ receptor deficient mice. Enlarged calluses were observed at 14, 21 and 28 days,

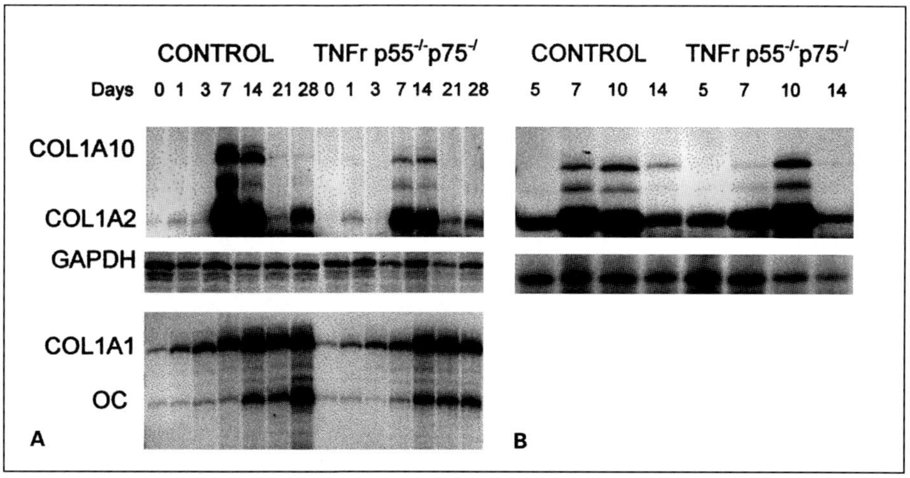

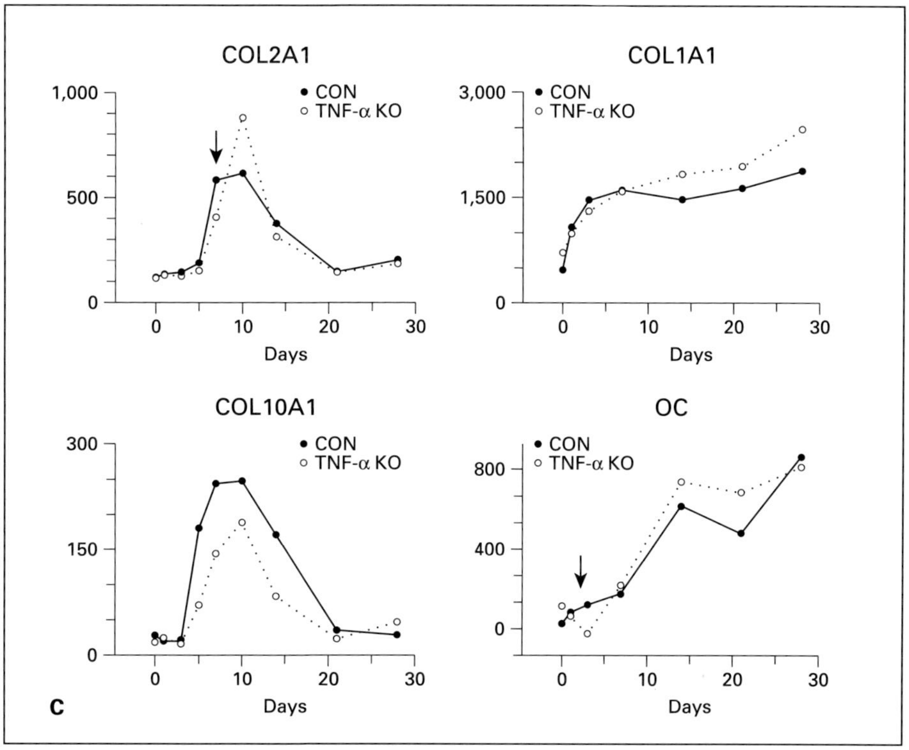

Fig. 2. Bone and cartilage gene expression during fracture repair in control and TNF-α receptor minus mice. **A**, **B** Representative RPA analysis of collagen types I, II, X, osteocalcin and GAPDH. Protections were carried out with 0.25 μg of total RNA and the protected mRNA templates were resolved on an 8% denaturing sequence gel. The times after fracture and the nature of the mice from which the mRNAs were obtained are denoted in the figure. **C** Graphic analysis of the relative mRNA levels. Band densities were determined from several different autoradiographic exposures. Band densities were normalized to the ratio of the internal standards, GAPDH and L32. Values represent the absolute quantities of each of the ECM genes. Arrows in COL2A1 and OC panels note the delays in and bone and cartilage induction.

and the bones were more fragile to being re-broke during dissection in the TNFR $p55^{-/-}/p75^{-/-}$ mice in comparison to the control animals. Histological analysis of the fracture sites confirmed the gross examination (fig. 1). The low magnification of the control and mutant animals at 21 days showed the enlarged nature of the calluses and a delay in removal of the calcified cartilage within the TNF-α receptor ablated mice. Higher magnification of the callus tissues at 200 × showed in detail the cellular alterations in the repair tissues at day 21. One of the most striking features of the histological examination was the delay in mesenchymal cell differentiation and the complete absence of the induction of the intramembranous bone formation on the periosteal surface. The failure to obtain intramembranous bone formation is better appreciated by comparison of the formation of an intramembranous bone bridge across the fracture gap seen in normal animals at 21 days compared to the lack of trabecular bridging seen at comparable post fracture times in the mutant animals (fig. 1, arrows). The delay in endochondral differentiation of the cartilage at later times was exemplified by the greater amounts of cartilage formed that were seen in

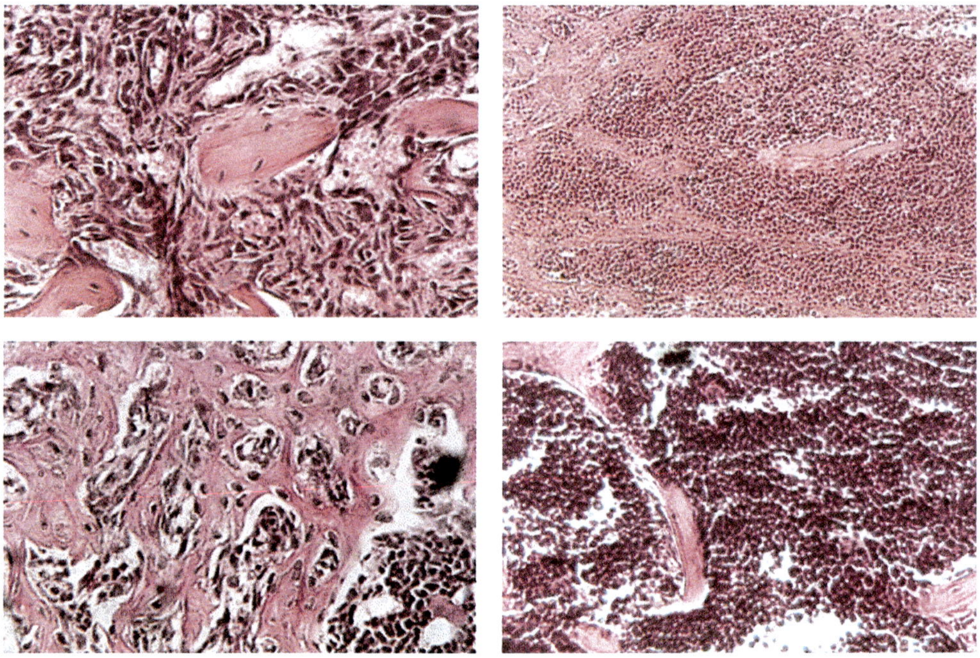

Fig. 3. Selected histological analysis of bone repair of wild-type (control) mice after marrow ablation. Days after marrow ablation are indicated in the figure. Low 40 × magnification panoramic view of the bone repair at days 1, 3, 7, 21 and 28. Note the high degree of cellularity in the control tibia marrow space and lack of trabecular bone. At 1 day, newly formed bone is readily apparent after marrow ablation, while by day 7, the marrow space is completely filled with newly formed trabecular bone. At days 21 and 28, the newly made bone is remodeling and the marrow space is being restored.

the callus and a delay in its hypertrophic maturation and removal in the mutant animals. Interestingly, at later times, even though intramembranous bone formation was absent in the mutant animals, there were a considerable number of osteogenic cells lining the cartilage tissue surfaces within the callus tissue.

The molecular processes of chondrocyte and osteoblast differentiation were assessed by analyzing the mRNA expression of various extracellular matrix gene products that are associated with the development of these tissues (fig. 2). These results demonstrated that the initial induction of bone formation, as exemplified by the expression of type I collagen and osteocalcin mRNA expression, was delayed but at later times the overall levels of these mRNAs were slightly higher (~20%) in the callus tissues from the mutant animals. The expression of collagen type II and X genes that are associated with growth and hypertrophic chondrocyte development, respectively, showed overall slightly lower levels of expression at the two time points that were initially examined (fig. 2, left panel). While this initial examination appeared to be inconsistent with the histological findings in figure 1, examination of a much narrower temporal window between days 5 and 14 (fig. 2, right panel) when the endochondral process is maximally occurring better showed the delay and the elevated levels of type II collagen expression at day 10. The retarded progression of hypertrophic development is easily seen in the shift in peak mRNA expression seen for type II collagen and the altered ratios of collagen type II to type X mRNA expression (fig. 2B). These results overall then confirmed at a molecular level the delay in the endochondral progression during fracture healing in the absence of TNF-α signaling.

In order to determine if the absence of TNF-α signaling has a direct effect on osteogenesis, bone repair was next examined in the marrow ablation model. In this model,

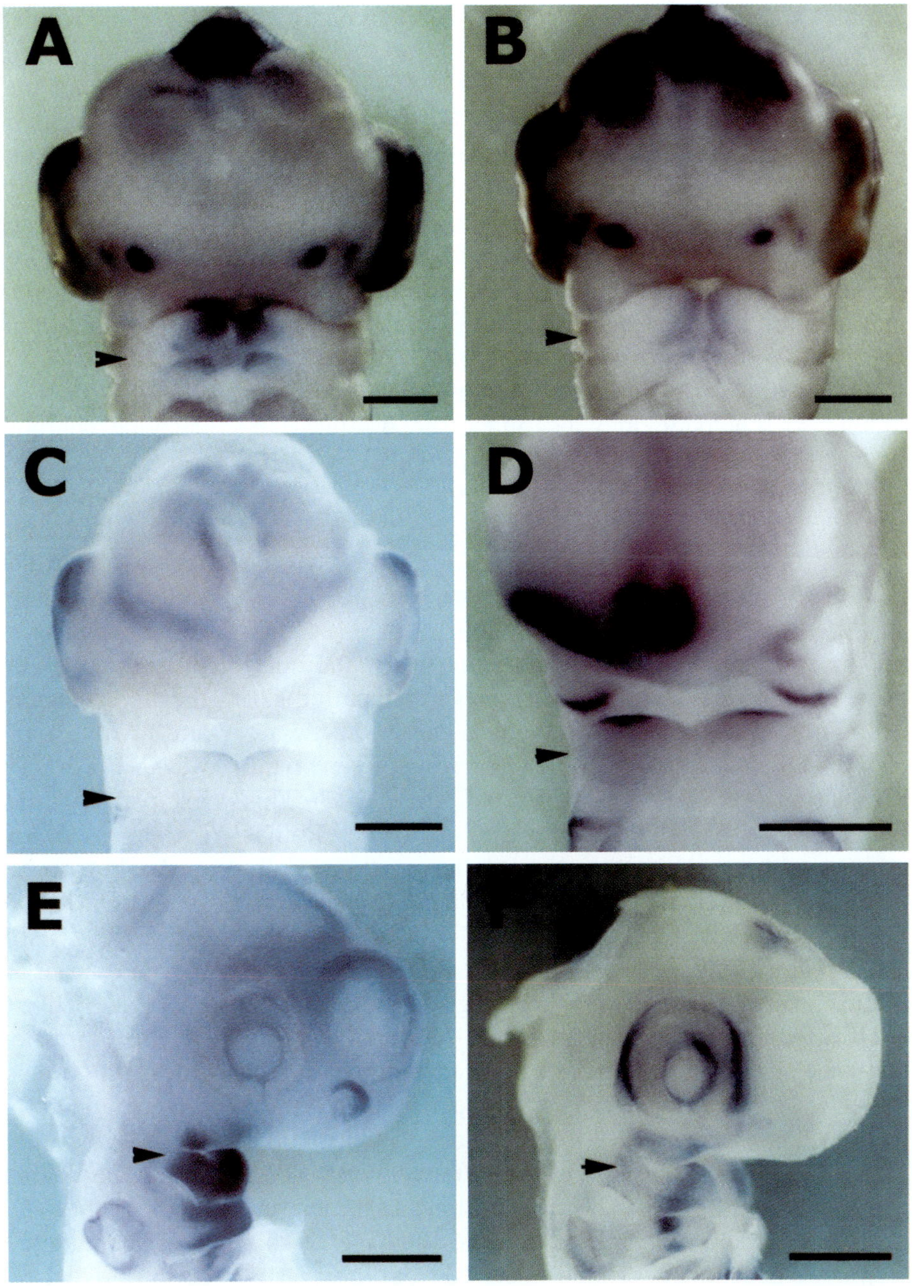

Fig. 1. Distribution of *Msx1* (**A**), *Msx2* (**B**), *Bmp4* (**C**), *Fgf8* (**D**), *Dlx5* (**E**), and *Wnt5a* (**F**) transcripts in whole mount preparations of stage chick face. **A–D** Frontal views. **E**, **F** Lateral views. Regions in which probes have hybridized are stained purple/blue. At stage 23, *Msx1* (**A**) and *Msx2* (**B**) are expressed in the medial region of the developing mandible. At stage 23, *Bmp4* (**C**) expression is restricted to the epithelium of the medial region, whereas *Fgf8* (**D**) is expressed in the epithelium covering the lateral regions of the developing mandible. Note the strong hybridization signals for *Dlx5* (**E**) and *Wnt5a* (**F**) in the mesenchyme of the lateral regions at stage 20. Arrowheads indicate the mandibular arch. Scale bars = 500 μm.

the interactions that regulate survival, outgrowth, and morphogenesis of the lateral regions [Trumpp et al., 1999]. In the mandible of newborn mutants in which *Fgf8* was inactivated in the epithelium of the first branchial arch using Cre/lox technology (*Fgf8;Nes-cre* mutants) skeletal elements in the lateral regions including the body of Meckel's cartilage, mandibular bones, molar teeth, and middle ear (except for malleus) were absent [Trumpp et al., 1999]. However, in these mutants the symphysial portion of Meckel's cartilage and the mandibular incisors and their associated bones were invariably present [Trumpp et al., 1999].

Studies in the chick mandible indicate that BMPs play stage-specific roles in apoptosis and chondrogenesis of the lateral regions [Barlow and Fancis-West, 1997; Ekanayake and Hall, 1997; Wang et al., 1999; Mina et al., 2000]. At early stages of development (stage 20) exogenous BMPs applied to the lateral region caused apoptosis, ectopic expression of *Msx* genes and inhibited outgrowth of the mandibular primordia and the formation of Meckel's cartilage [Barlow and Francis-West, 1997; Ekanayake and Hall, 1997; Mina et al., 2000]. On the other hand, treatment at stage 23 resulted in the formation of ectopic cartilage in the caudal region of Meckel's cartilage [Barlow and Francis-West, 1997; Wang et al., 1999]. These observations on the apoptotic effects of BMPs in the lateral mandibular mesenchyme where survival of mesenchymal cells and morphogenesis has been shown to be dependent on FGF-8-mediated signaling [Trumpp et al., 1999] suggest that at early stages of development lateral mandibular mesenchyme may be under the balanced influence of death and survival signals provided by BMPs and FGFs respectively [Mina et al., 2000].

Morphogenesis of the Medial Region

The small medial region, where the two mandibular processes merge, is characterized by restricted patterns of expression of *Bmp4* in the epithelium and *Msx1, Msx2, HAND, Bmp2,* and *Fgfr2* in the underlying mesenchyme [Francis-West et al., 1998; Mina, 2000] (fig. 1A–C). This region gives rise to the medial region of the mandibular arch containing incisor teeth, and the most medially located skeletal elements including the symphysial portion of Meckel's cartilage.

Available evidence suggests that the medial region is a putative signaling center that plays a significant role in the outgrowth of the developing mandible. The medial region contains highly proliferative mesenchymal cells and makes a significant contribution to the overall growth of the developing mandible [Richman and Tickle, 1989; Mina et al., 1995, 2000; Barlow and Francis-West, 1997; McGonnell et al., 1998]. The proliferation and the expression of a number of genes in the mesenchyme of this region are dependent on signals derived from the overlying epithelium [Francis-West et al., 1999; Mina, 2000].

The lack of abnormalities in the medial region in *Fgf8;Nes-cre* mutants provides clear evidence that, unlike the lateral region, the small medial region depends on signals other than FGF-8 [Trumpp et al., 1999] and leaves open the question of which signal(s) are involved in morphogenesis of this region. The available evidence suggests that morphogenesis of the medial region is regulated by multiple signaling pathways.

The unchanged patterns of expression of markers of the medial region, including *Bmp-4, dHAND, eHAND, Msx1,* and *Msx2* in *Fgf8;Nes-cre* mutant embryos suggest that these regulatory molecules are involved in morphogenesis of the medial region [Trumpp et al., 1999]. The possibility of the involvement of *Msx1* and *dHAND* in morphogenesis of the medial region is supported by the abnormalities in the medial region of mice deficient for *Msx1* or *dHAND* [Satokata and Maas, 1994; Thomas et al., 1998; Srivastava, 1999].

In addition to *Msx1* and *dHAND* mutant mice, mice lacking other regulatory genes including genes encoding components of the endothelin pathway *(ETA, ET1, ECE-1)* [Kurihara et al., 1999], *Wnt5a* [Yamaguchi et al., 1999], *Pitx2* [Lin et al., 1999; Lu et al., 1999b], and mice carrying compound mutations in *Prx1* and *Prx2* [ten Berge et al., 1998; Lu et al., 1999a] all exhibit a subset of abnormalities in the medial region of the developing mandible. The shared subset of abnormalities in the medial region of the developing mandible in various mutants indicates the essential roles of these gene products for correct morphogenesis of the medial region and suggests that the regulatory hierarchies controlling morphogenesis of the medial region of the developing mandible are complex and involve many molecules and possibly multiple pathways. However, it is currently not clear how many signaling pathways regulate the development of the medial region.

Analyses of *dHAND–/–, ETA–/–,* and *ET1–/–* mutants provide information for one of the genetic pathways, the 'ET-1-dHAND-Msx1 pathway', that is involved in morphogenesis of the medial region of the mandible [Thomas et al., 1998; Clouthier et al., 2000].

The expression of a number of other signaling molecules and transcription factors in the epithelium and mesenchyme of the medial region [Mina, 2000] are also suggestive of their roles in morphogenesis of the medial region. Based on their patterns of expression, members of the BMP and FGF families of signaling molecules are also likely candidates involved in regulating morphogenesis of the medial region [Francis-West et al., 1998; Mina, 2000].

In the developing mandible multiple *Bmp* genes are expressed by the epithelium of the medial region [Francis-West et al., 1998; Mina, 2000]. Among these, *Bmp4* expression is restricted to the epithelium in the medial region [Francis-West et al., 1994; Wang et al., 1998] and is not affected in the mandibles of *Fgf8;Nes-cre* mutants [Trumpp et al., 1999]. BMPs are capable of inducing *Msx1* and *Msx2* expression in a variety of mesenchymes including chick and mouse mandibular mesenchyme [Francis-West et al., 1998, No. 26; Mina, 2000]. Roles for BMP-4 in morphogenesis of the medial region are supported by the finding that inhibition of BMP signaling in this region results in downregulation of *Msx1*, ectopic expression of *Barx1* and changes in tooth morphogenesis such that molar teeth develop in place of incisors [Tucker et al., 1998b].

The possible involvement of BMPs in signaling pathways regulating the growth of the branchial arches is supported by phenotypic abnormalities in the *Bmp5/Bmp7* double knockout [Solloway and Robertson, 1999]. Analysis of *Bmp5/Bmp7* mutants revealed abnormalities in development of many organs including the developing mandibular arches where *Bmp5* and *Bmp7* are coexpressed. The mandibles in double mutants were smaller than those in the wild type, and displayed increased apoptosis in the surface ectoderm at the base of the first branchial arch and defects in the mesodermally derived mesenchyme. These observations suggest that these BMPs secreted by mandibular epithelium may be required for maintenance/survival of mesodermally derived cells in the mandible [Solloway and Robertson, 1999].

Studies in the ckick mandible indicate that BMPs can mimic many of the effects of mandibular epithelium from the medial region on the mandibular mesenchyme [Barlow and Francis-West, 1997; Wang et al., 1998b, 1999; Mina et al., 2000]. However, unlike mandibular epithelium, medially placed BMPs do not support the elongation of mandibular mesenchyme and Meckel's cartilage [Wang et al., 1999; Mina et al., 2000]. Since BMPs are unable to support the full outgrowth of the mandibular mesenchyme, it remains unclear whether BMPs are involved in mediating the growth promoting effects of mandibular epithelium on the underlying mesenchyme [Wang et al., 1999].

On the other hand, unlike their apoptotic effects on the undifferentiated mesenchyme of the lateral region [Barlow and Francis-West, 1997; Ekanayake and Hall, 1997; Mina et al., 2000], beads soaked in BMPs implanted in vivo to medial region of mandible of stage 20 (but not stage 23) induced the formation of a well-organized duplicated rod of cartilage extending from the body of Meckel's cartilage [Barlow and Francis-West, 1997; Mina et al., 2000]. The formation of ectopic cartilage by medially (stage 20) and laterally (stage 23) placed BMP beads is consistent with the roles of BMP-mediated signaling in the multistep process of chondrogenesis of the mandibular mesenchyme.

Functional studies suggest that FGFs secreted by the epithelium of the medial region are part of the signaling pathway regulating mandibular outgrowth [Richman et al., 1997; Mina et al., 2000]. In the absence of epithelium, FGF beads placed on the mesenchyme of the medial region (but not mesenchyme of the lateral regions) can support the expression of *Msx* genes, outgrowth of the mandibular processes and elongation of Meckel's cartilage [Richman et al., 1997; Mina et al., 2000]. Based on expression patterns, FGFs other than FGF-8 that are secreted by epithelium of the medial region including FGF-2 and FGF-4 are likely endogenous signals involved in growth of the medial region of the mandible [Richman et al., 1997; Mina, 2000; Mina et al., 2000]. FGFs transmit their signals through several different types of receptors including the four high-affinity transmembrane receptors that are designated FGFR1–4 [Szebenyi and Fallon, 1999; Kannan and Givol, 2000]. Among these, *Fgfr2* is the only *Fgfr* that is expressed in the mesenchyme of the medial region [Orr-Urtreger et al., 1991; Wilke et al., 1997; Mina et al., 2000]. An interesting feature of this family of receptors is the existence of numerous mRNA isoforms generated by alternative splicing [Szebenyi and Fallon, 1999; Kannan and Givol, 2000]. For example, alternative splicing of exons 8 and 9 of *Fgfr2* results in the generation of IIIb (*Fgfr2b* containing exon 8) and IIIc (*Fgfr2c* containing exon 9) isoforms with different ligand specificities and different tissue distributions [Szebenyi and Fallon, 1999; Kannan and Givol, 2000]. It has been shown in many organs that *Fgfr2c* is expressed mainly by mesenchyme and is activated by FGF-1, FGF-2, FGF-4, FGF-6, and FGF-9 [Ornitz et al., 1996; Szebenyi and Fallon, 1999; Kannan and Givol, 2000]. Despite the lack of information about isoform-specific patterns of expression *Fgfr2c* and *Fgfr2b* in the developing mandible, the mesenchymal localization in other organs suggests that in the developing mandible FGFR2c mediates the effects of FGF signals originating from the epithelium of the medial region on the underlying mesenchyme. However, understanding the roles of this pathway in mandibular morphogenesis through standard gene targeting approaches has been problematic. A null mutation encompassing both isoforms of *Fgfr2* results in pre-implantation lethality [Arman et al., 1998] and mice expressing a hypomorphic allele of Fgfr2 die around E10 [Xu et al., 1998]. However, mutant animals specifically deficient for the *Egfr2b* isoform and mice expressing a soluble dominant negative form of *Egfr2b* had cleft palate, smaller faces and abnormalities in many tissues where morphogenesis is dependent on epithelial-mesenchymal interactions [Celli et al., 1998; De Moerlooze et al., 2000].

In addition to expressing *Bmps, ET-1,* and *Fgfs,* mandibular epithelium also expresses other regulatory genes including *Jagged2, Pitx2, PDGFA,* and *Egf* and *Egfr*

[Francis-West et al., 1998; Mina, 2000]. The roles of some of these gene products in the outgrowth and morphogenesis of the mandibular arch have also been elucidated by phenotypic abnormalities in knockouts [Soriano, 1997; Sidow et al., 1997; Miettinen et al., 1999; Lin et al., 1999; Lu et al., 1999b].

Conclusions

Elucidating the molecular pathways and mechanisms regulating development and morphogenesis of the mandibular arch is fundamental to understanding the pathogenesis of the numerous human congenital syndromes which manifest severe abnormalities in first branchial arch derivatives including first arch syndromes, Treacher-Collins syndrome and Pierre Robin sequence. Abnormalities in the mandibles of various mouse mutants caused by targeted inactivation of individual candidate molecules and compound mutants provide powerful tools for examining the hierarchy of signaling molecules involved in mandibular morphogenesis. Furthermore, accessibility of the developing face in the chick embryo for experimental manipulations, and detailed analysis of chick mutants with abnormalities in the lower jaw will continue to provide invaluable information in the area of craniofacial biology.

Acknowledgments

The author wishes to thank Dr. Y.-H. Wang for preparing figure 1. The work in the author's laboratory was supported by NIH Grant DE08682.

References

Arman, E., R. Haffner-Krausz, Y. Chen, J.K. Heath, P. Lonai (1998) Targeted disruption of fibroblast growth factor (FGF) receptor 2 suggests a role for FGF signaling in pregastrulation mammalian development. Proc Natl Acad Sci USA *95:* 5082–5087.

Barlow, A.J., P.H. Francis-West (1997) Ectopic application of recombinant BMP-2 and BMP-4 can change patterning of developing chick facial primordia. Development *124:* 391–398.

Celli, G., W.J. LaRochelle, S. Mackem, R. Sharp, G. Merlino (1998) soluble dominant-negative receptor uncovers essential roles for fibroblast growth factors in multi-organ induction and patterning. EMBO J *17:* 1642–1655.

Chai, Y., X. Jiang, Y. Ito, P. Bringas, J. Han , D.H. Rowitch, P. Soriano, A.P. McMahon, H.M. Sucov (2000) Fate of the mammalian cranial neural crest during tooth and mandibular morphogenesis (in process citation). Development *127:* 1671–1679.

Clouthier, D.E., S.C. Williams, H. Yanagisawa, M. Wieduwilt, J.A. Richardson, M. Yanagisawa (2000) Signaling pathways crucial for craniofacial development revealed by endothelin-A receptor-deficient mice. Dev Biol *217:* 10–24.

Couly, G., A. Grapin-Botton, P. Coltey, N.M. Le Douarin (1996) The regeneration of the cephalic neural crest, a problem revisited: The regenerating cells originate from the contralateral or from the anterior and posterior neural fold. Development *122:* 3393–3407.

Couly, G., A. Grapin-Botton, P. Coltey, B. Ruhin, N.M. Le Douarin (1998) Determination of the identity of the derivatives of the cephalic neural crest: Incompatibility between Hox gene expression and lower jaw development. Development *125:* 3445–3459.

Couly, G.F., P.M. Coltey, N.M. Le Douarin (1992) The developmental fate of the cephalic mesoderm in quail-chick chimeras. Development *114:* 1–15.

Couly, G.F., P.M. Coltey, N.M. Le Douarin (1993) The triple origin of skull in higher vertebrates: a study in quail-chick chimeras. Development *117:* 409–429.

De Moerlooze, L., B. Spencer-Dene, J. Revest, M. Hajihosseini, I. Rosewell, C. Dickinson (2000) An important role for the IIIb isoform of fibroblast growth factor receptor 2 (FGFR2) in mesenchymal-epithelial signalling during mouse organogenesis (in process citation). Development *127:* 483–492.

Ekanayake, S., B.K. Hall (1997) The in vivo and in vitro effects of bone morphogenetic protein-2 on the development of the chick mandible. Int J Dev Biol *41:* 67–81.

Ferguson, C.A., A.S. Tucker, P.T. Sharpe (2000) Temporospatial cell interactions regulating mandibular and maxillary arch patterning. Development *127:* 403–412.

Francis-West, P., R. Ladher, A. Barlow, A. Graveson (1998) Signaling interactions during facial development. Mech Dev *75:* 3–28.

Francis-West, P.H., T. Tatla, P.M. Brickell (1994) Expression patterns of the bone morphogenetic protein genes Bmp-4 and Bmp-2 in the developing chick face suggest a role in outgrowth of the primordia. Dev Dyn *201:* 168–178.

Hacker, A., S. Guthrie (1998) A distinct developmental programme for the cranial paraxial mesoderm in the chick embryo. Development *125:* 3461–3472.

Kannan, K., D. Givol (2000) FGF receptor mutations: Dimerization syndromes, cell growth suppression, and animal models. IUBMB Life *49:* 197–205.

Kontges, G., A. Lumsden (1996) Rhombencephalic neural crest segmentation is preserved throughout craniofacial ontogeny. Development *122:* 3229–3242.

Kurihara, H., Y. Kurihara, R. Nagai, Y. Yazaki (1999) Endothelin and neural crest development. Cell Mol Biol *45:* 639–651.

Lin, C.R., C. Kioussi, S. O'Connell, P. Briata, D. Szeto, F. Liu, J.C. Izpisua-Belmonte, M.G. Rosenfeld (1999) Pitx2 regulates lung asymmetry, cardiac positioning and pituitary and tooth morphogenesis. Nature *401:* 279–282.

Lu, M.F., H.T. Cheng, M.J. Kern, S.S. Potter, B. Tran, T.G. Diekwisch, J.F. Martin (1999a) prx-1 functions cooperatively with another paired-related homeobox gene, prx-2, to maintain cell fates within the craniofacial mesenchyme. Development *126:* 495–504.

Lu, M.F., H.T. Cheng, A.R. Lacy, M.J. Kern, E.A. Argao, S.S. Potter, E.N. Olson, J.F. Martin (1999b) Paired-related homeobox genes cooperate in handplate and hindlimb zeugopod morphogenesis. Dev Biol *205:* 145–157.

Mallo, M. (1998) Embryological and genetic aspects of middle ear development. Int J Dev Biol *42:* 11–22.

McGonnell, I.M., J.D. Clarke, C. Tickle (1998) Fate map of the developing chick face: Analysis of expansion of facial primordia and establishment of the primary palate. Dev Dyn *212:* 102–118.

Miettinen, P.J., J.R. Chin, L. Shum, H.C. Slavkin, C.F. Shuler, R. Derynck, Z. Werb (1999) Epidermal growth factor receptor function is necessary for normal craniofacial development and palate closure. Nat Genet *22:* 69–73.

Mina, M. (2000) Regulation of mandibular growth and morphogenesis: Critical review. Oral Biol Med, in press.

Mina, M., J. Gluhak, W.B. Upholt, E.J. Kollar, B. Rogers (1995) Experimental analysis of Msx-1 and Msx-2 gene expression during chick mandibular morphogenesis. Dev Dyn *202:* 195–214.

Mina, M., Y.-H. Wang, A.M. Ivanovics, B. Rodgers (2000) Region- and stage-specific effects of FGFs and BMPs in chick mandibular morphogenesis. Submitted.

Neubuser, A., H. Peters, R. Balling, G.R. Martin (1997) Antagonistic interactions between FGF and BMP signaling pathways: A mechanism for positioning the sites of tooth formation. Cell *90:* 247–255.

Noden, D.M. (1983) The embryonic origins of avian cephalic and cervical muscles and associated connective tissues. Am J Anat *168:* 257–276.

Ornitz, D.M., J. Xu, J.S. Colvin, D.G. McEwen, C.A. MacArthur, F. Coulier, G. Gao, M. Goldfarb (1996) Receptor specificity of the fibroblast growth factor family. J Biol Chem *271:* 15292–15297.

Orr-Urtreger, A., D. Givol, A. Yayon, Y. Yarden, P. Lonai (1991) Developmental expression of two murine fibroblast growth factor receptors, flg and bek. Development *113:* 1419–1434.

Osumi-Yamashita, N., Y. Ninomiya, K. Eto (1997) Mammalian craniofacial embryology in vitro. Int J Dev Biol *41:* 187–194.

Richman, J.M., M. Herbert, E. Matovinovic, J. Walin (1997) Effect of fibroblast growth factors on outgrowth of facial mesenchyme. Dev Biol *189:* 135–147.

Richman, J.M., C. Tickle (1989) Epithelia are interchangeable between facial primordia of chick embryos and morphogenesis is controlled by the mesenchyme. Dev Biol *136:* 201–210.

Satokata, I., R. Maas (1994) Msx1 deficient mice exhibit cleft palate and abnormalities of craniofacial and tooth development. Nat Genet *6:* 348–356.

Sidow, A., M.S. Bulotsky, A.W. Kerrebrock, R.T. Bronson, M.J. Daly, M.P. Reeve, T.L. Hawkins, B.W. Birren, R. Jaenisch, E.S. Lander (1997) Serrate2 is disrupted in the mouse limb-development mutant syndactylism. Nature *389:* 722–725.

Sohal, G.S., M.M. Ali, A.A. Ali, D. Dai (1999) Ventrally emigrating neural tube cells contribute to the formation of Meckel's and quadrate cartilage. Dev Dyn *216:* 37–44.

Soriano, P. (1997) The PDGF alpha receptor is required for neural crest cell development and for normal patterning of the somites. Development *124:* 2691–2700.

Srivastava, D. (1999) HAND proteins: Molecular mediators of cardiac development and congenital heart disease. Trends Cardiovasc Med *9:* 11–18.

Szebenyi, G., J.F. Fallon (1999) Fibroblast growth factors as multifunctional signaling factors. Int Rev Cytol *185:* 45–106.

ten Berge, D., A. Brouwer, J. Korving, J.F. Martin, F. Meijlink (1998) Prx1 and Prx2 in skeletogenesis: roles in the craniofacial region, inner ear and limbs. Development *125:* 3831–3842.

Thomas, T., H. Kurihara, H. Yamagishi, Y. Kurihara, Y. Yazaki, E.N. Olson, D. Srivastava (1998) A signaling cascade involving endothelin-1, dHAND and msx1 regulates development of neural-crest-derived brancihal arch mesenchyme. Development *125:* 3005–3014.

Trainor, P.A., P.P. Tam (1995) Cranial paraxial mesoderm and neural crest cells of the mouse embryo: co-distribution in the craniofacial mesenchyme but distinct segregation in branchial arches. Development *121:* 2569–2582.

Trainor, P.A., S.S. Tan, P.P. Tam (1994) Cranial paraxial mesoderm: regionalisation of cell fate and impact on craniofacial development in mouse embryos. Development *120:* 2397–2408.

Trumpp, A., M.J. Depew, J.L. Rubenstein, J.M. Bishop, G.R. Martin (1999) Cre-mediated gene inactivation demonstrates that FGF8 is required for cell survival and patterning of the first branchial arch. Genes Dev *13:* 3136–3148.

Tucker, A.S., A. Al Khamis, P.T. Sharpe (1998a) Interactions between Bmp-4 and Msx-1 act to restrict gene expression to odontogenic mesenchyme. Dev Dyn *212:* 533–539.

Tucker, A.S., K.L. Matthews, P.T. Sharpe (1998b) Transformation of tooth type induced by inhibition of BMP signaling. Science *282:* 1136–1138.

Wang, Y.H., B. Rutherford, W.B. Upholt, M. Mina (1999) Effects of BMP-7 on mouse tooth mesenchyme and chick mandibular mesenchyme. Dev Dyn *216:* 320–335.

Wang, Y.H., W.B. Upholt, P.T. Sharpe, E.J. Kollar, M. Mina (1998) Odontogenic epithelium induces similar molecular responses in chick and mouse mandibular mesenchyme. Dev Dyn *213:* 386–397.

Wilke, T.A., S. Gubbels, J. Schwartz, J.M. Richman (1997) Expression of fibroblast growth factor receptors (FGFR1, FGFR2, FGFR3) in the developing head and face. Dev Dyn *210:* 41–52.

Xu, X., M. Weinstein, C. Li, M. Naski, R.I. Cohen, D.M. Ornitz , P. Leder, C. Deng (1998) Fibroblast growth factor receptor 2 (FGFR2)-mediated reciprocal regulation loop between FGF8 and FGF10 is essential for limb induction. Development *125:* 753–765.

Yamaguchi, T.P., A. Bradley, A.P. McMahon, S. Jones (1999) A Wnt5a pathway underlies outgrowth of multiple structures in the vertebrate embryo. Development *126:* 1211–1223.

Cells
Tissues
Organs

Cells Tissues Organs 2001;169:302–308

Engineered Cartilage, Bone, Joints, and Menisci

Potential for Temporomandibular Joint Reconstruction

Julie Glowacki

Orthopedic Research, Brigham and Women's Hospital, Harvard Medical School, and Skeletal Biology Research Center, Massachusetts General Hospital, Harvard School of Dental Medicine, Boston, Mass., USA

Key Words
Tissue engineering · Temporomandibular joint · Meniscus · Cartilage · Bone

Abstract
Reconstruction of many musculoskeletal structures can be accomplished by bone grafting and implantation of prostheses. Alternate approaches are needed, however, for repair of complex structures such as articular cartilage surfaces and the temporomandibular meniscus and joint. Tissue engineering, either cell-free or cell-based, offers promise because of recent advances in materials research and in our knowledge of the cellular and molecular mechanisms of tissue repair. There are three considerations in designing a construct for engineered tissue: the source of cells, if any; the nature of the carrier or scaffold; and use, if any, of genes, factors, or adjuvants. Autogenous cells, often expanded in vitro, have been useful for cartilage tissue engineering. Precursor/progenitor cells are advantageous for bone tissue. There are many natural and synthetic resorbable materials with good biocompatibility and tissue compatibility that can be modified to have the porosity and mechanical properties needed for specific applications. The scaffolds can also be modified to provide biological signals to augment repair and integration.

Introduction

Skeletal deficiencies due to congenital or acquired pathology can be managed by various prevailing surgical procedures including transplantation of freshly harvested autogenous bone, bone distraction and segment transport, implantation of banked allogenic tissues, and use of alloplastic bone-substitute materials. In contrast to bone, severely damaged and deformed articular cartilage surfaces in hips, knees, and hands are generally not amenable to focal treatments, usually requiring replacement of the entire joint with metal prostheses. Even fewer options are available for severe deformities of the temporomandibular joint (TMJ). Clinical advances with cell-based therapies and experimental progress with engineered scaffolds and constructs raise the possibility that novel approaches may become more widely available, perhaps even in early stages of degeneration.

There are two major engineering approaches to novel treatments of bone and joint problems: cell-based and cell-free (fig. 1). In both, materials are engineered to provide optimum function for specific applications. Simply put, scaffolds for cell-based therapies are intended to provide a compatible carrier for viable cells for enhanced histogenesis, function, and integration with the recipient tissue bed. Scaffolds for cell-free repair are designed to stimulate neohistogenesis, often by mimicking signals for ana-

KARGER

Fax + 41 61 306 12 34
E-Mail karger@karger.ch
www.karger.com

Accessible online at:
www.karger.com/journals/cto

Julie Glowacki, PhD
Orthopedic Surgery, Brigham and Women's Hospital
75 Francis Street
Boston, MA 02115 (USA)
Tel. +1 617 732 5397, Fax +1 617 732 6937

bolic processes (called biomimetic implants). Either may contain genes, factors, or adjuvants to promote the desired pathway and inhibit undesired processes. Chemical and geometric properties of scaffold materials are critical for cell viability, for production of matrix, and for in vivo compatibility (table 1). Major classes of biocompatible scaffolds include natural and synthetic polymers and ceramics [Ratner et al., 1996; Lanza et al., 1997]. The polymers have been especially useful supports for engineered cartilage [Glowacki, 2000; Temenoff and Mikos, 2000]; whereas the ceramics and glasses have been evaluated for bone [Mueller and Glowacki, 2000]. Injectable carriers, notably those that polymerize or solidify in vivo, may be useful for percutaneous management of small lesions. For integration with the recipient bed, solid scaffolds need to be resorbable or should have a porosity or woven form or favorable texture. Interest in 'smart' scaffolds concerns surface modifications to promote favorable interactions with seeded cells and/or host tissues. Coatings and adsorption or activation with bioactive molecules can also improve performance [Boyan et al., 1999]. These principles have been applied with varying success for musculoskeletal repair and reconstruction, but opportunities exist for novel procedures.

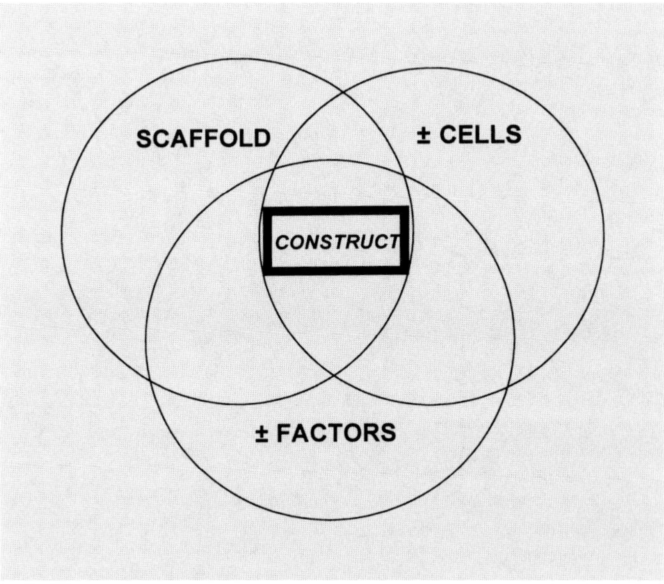

Fig. 1. Schematic for design of tissue engineered construct. The scaffold, either resorbable or permanent, may serve three functions: as an engineered material for implantation and ingrowth of needed tissue; as a carrier for cells that have been freshly obtained or expanded in vitro; or as a delivery system for genes, factors, or drugs. Cells may be seeded prior to implantation of the construct. Factors (e.g. peptide coatings, genes, growth factors, angiogenic factors, antibiotics) can be incorporated into and/or delivered from the construct.

Cartilage

Adult human cartilage shows poor capacity for repair and regeneration, thus requiring innovative solutions for congenital, traumatic, and degenerative cartilage lesions. Cartilage has been a model for research of in vitro engineered tissues because it is a relatively simple tissue with respect to its cellular homogeneity and avascularity.

Clinical advances have been made since Grande et al.'s [1989] landmark report on autologous chondrocyte transplantation for experimental defects in rabbits. In a 3-step process [Brittberg et al., 1994], normal cartilage is first harvested from a nonbearing part of the knee. Next, cells are isolated and expanded in vitro. In a second surgical procedure, the lesion is prepared and covered with a fresh periosteal patch beneath which a suspension of the expanded cells is delivered. Other approaches for simplifying the delivery and ensuring the retention of the cells include the use of a scaffold.

Some of the problems with chondrocyte expansion and in vitro chondrogenesis concern the limited expansion potential for adult cells, general nutritional unknowns, and optimization of culture conditions. There are many ways to influence growth and function of cells in vitro.

Table 1. Some characteristics of scaffolds for tissue engineering

Composition
Natural polymers (collagen, hyaluronan, fibrin, alginates, silks)
Synthetic polymers
Resorbable (poly[lactide-co-glycolide], polycarbonates)
Permanent (PMMA)
Ceramics (calcium phosphates), glasses
Form
Injectable
Polymerize, solidify
Solid, gel, solution
Crystalline, amorphous, biphasic
Fibers, particles
Porosity
Modifications
Surface texture, patterning
Adsorbed, immobilized molecules
Coatings, adjuvants, composite, reinforced
Delivery of genes, factors, drugs

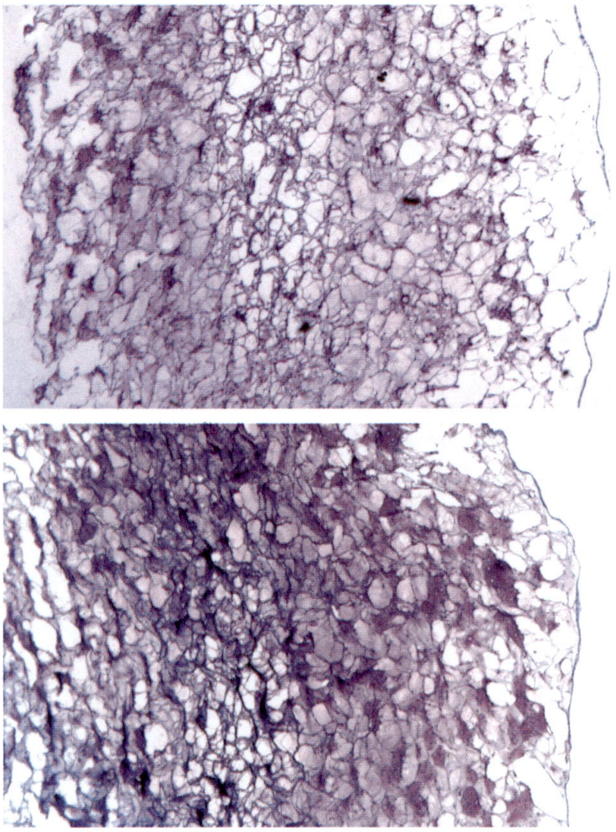

Fig. 2. Photomicrograph of 3-dimensional collagen sponge cultured for 7 days (upper) and 14 days (lower) with bovine articular chondrocytes. The surfaces of the sponges are on the right side. Metachromatic extracellular matrix accumulated throughout the sponges. Foci of dense cartilage are especially evident in lower, right.

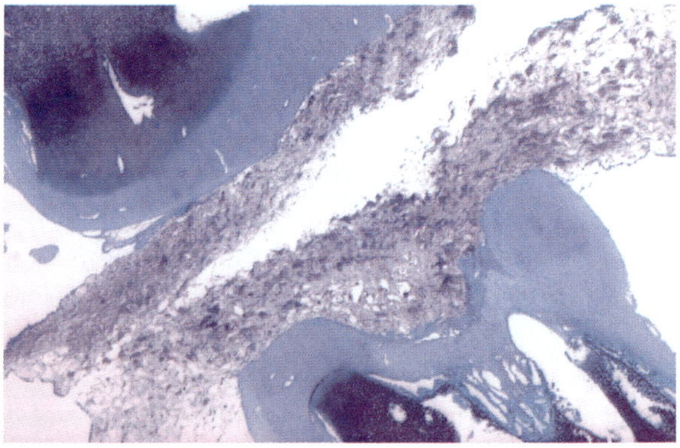

Fig. 3. Photomicrograph of chimeric construct of bovine articular chondrocytes seeded in two 3-D collagen sponges and inserted into a devitalized embryonic chick knee. One week after incubation, the construct shows accumulation of extracellular matrix and fusion of the collagen sponges with host articular surfaces.

Supplementation with chondrocyte growth and differentiation factors is useful, the 3-D format is superior to monolayer culture for differentiated activities [Allemann et al., 2000], and chondrogenesis is enhanced at low oxygen concentrations [Mizuno and Glowacki, 2000]. Mechanical factors are also important for in vitro chondrogenesis; for example, Mizuno et al. [1997] reported that hydrostatic fluid pressure stimulated chondrogenesis in 3-D collagen sponges.

There are various scaffolds or vehicles that have been used for chondrocytes [Glowacki, 2000]. Devitalized cartilage matrix itself was used with fibrin as a substrate for neochondrogenesis by isolated chondrocytes [Peretti et al, 1998]. Collagen [Mizuno and Glowacki, 1996] and other natural polymers can be made as porous 3-D carriers for chondrocytes (fig. 2). We recently reported that addition of hyaluronan into the collagen scaffold enhanced the extent of chondrogenesis [Allemann et al., 2001]. These show excellent integration with host tissues. Various synthetic polymers, mostly resorbable ones, are also being developed for reconstruction [Vacanti et al., 1991]. They have the advantage of plentiful supply and precise control of composition and possibilities of resorbable features.

In the current clinical protocol, normal autogenous cells are used [Brittberg et al., 1994]. As alternatives to these and the requisite damage in harvesting normal cartilage, marrow-derived cells have been shown to have potential for chondrocytic differentiation [Wakitani et al., 1994]. In another approach, we showed that human skin fibroblasts can be stimulated to produce cartilage matrix in 3-D collagen scaffolds that contain inductive demineralized bone powder [Mizuno and Glowacki, 1996; Glowacki et al., 1998b]. It is evident that integrated optimization of the source and number of chondrogenic cells, development of 'smart' scaffolds that convey important regulatory information to the engineered tissue, definition of the chemical and mechanical environment during the in vitro phase, and integration of neocartilage constructs with the recipient bed should provide more consistent functional tissue [Glowacki, 2000].

Bone

Similar issues exist for engineering bone: source of cells, nature of the carrier, and effects of regulatory factors or genes [Mueller and Glowacki, 2000]. Bone tissue engineering has additional demands that relate to the differences between cartilage and bone. Bone is a more rigid and vascularized tissue that is required to bear and adapt to great load.

There may be some advantage for at least some woven bone to have formed in vitro prior to transplantation. For cells with greater dependence on aerobic glycolysis than chondrocytes, high-density, micromass or 3-D cultures have the problem of central necrosis. Control of, and monitoring of, culture conditions can maintain histogenesis in vitro for extended periods. For example, we reported that medium perfusion of 3-D cultures of murine osteoblasts enhanced viability and biosynthetic activity as assessed by osteoblastic phenotype and mineral deposition [Mueller et al., 1999]. Perfusion of medium through 3-D co-cultures of murine marrow stromal and hematopoietic cells enhanced their viability and differential functions [Glowacki et al., 1998a]. An additional element for osseous engraftment is the need for neovascularization. Cell and tissue viability may be at risk if neovascularization is too slow. If the bone formed in vitro is too dense, it may be difficult for small capillaries to invade it rapidly and efficiently. Thus it is likely that bone tissue formed during the in vitro stage would need to be implanted before the formation of very dense bone matrix [Mueller and Glowacki, 2000] or with supplemental angiogenic stimuli [Symes et al., 1999].

Adult bone-derived osteocytes and osteoblasts may not have sufficient growth potential for autogenous cell therapy. Bone marrow-derived cells contain precursor/progenitor cells that can be expanded in culture and used to engineer new bone [Friedenstein et al., 1966; Goshima et al., 1991].

For all of these reasons and the innate capacity of bone to regenerate, it is probable that cell-free systems may find more use for bone repair than for engineering of other organs. There has been some progress with the use of recombinant morphogens, like the BMPs, but long-term results need to be assessed [Boyne et al., 1997]. The solution for bone tissue may be the use of novel weight-bearing, biomimetic scaffolds that will enhance bone formation and angiogenesis in the space defined by the implant.

Joints

Although there has been success in the evolution of designs for orthopedic joint prostheses, the same cannot be said for complex structures like the mandibular condyle. Whether a cell-based or cell-free approach is wanted, modeling of the precise 3-D geometry of the joint structures will be required. Innovative approaches will be needed. To this end, Feinberg's group demonstrated the potential of an image-based system in which CT or MRI data directed a 3-dimensional fabrication machine to construct a scaffold for a mandibular condyle [Hollister et al., 2000].

There are alternatives to manufactured prostheses. Zaleske's group has proposed that a natural joint, once it has been devitalized and cleansed of antigens, has the potential to serve as a template for joint reconstruction [Caruso et al., 1996]. To that end, chondrocytes were shown to repopulate devitalized and perforated articular surfaces from the knees of embryonic chicks [Caruso et al., 1996]. Further, treatment of the joint with enzymes appeared to enhance chondrocytes' penetration into the devitalized cartilage matrix [Zaleske et al., 1999]. Recently, progress has been made in engineering a biological joint [Zaleske and Glowacki, unpubl. data]. Three-dimensional collagen scaffolds were used as an inert carrier of bovine articular chondrocytes [Mizuno and Glowacki, 1996]. One day after seeding, two of these sponges were inserted into a devitalized embryonic chick knee; after another week of incubation, the construct showed accumulation of matrix in the collagen sponges and integration with the underlying epiphyses (fig. 3). Pilot data suggest that the viable chondrocytes can invade the devitalized chick cartilage. This approach is based upon the hypothesis that cartilage matrix provides the structure for expansion of chondrocytes and the signals that chondrocytes recognize as native and favorable for growth and function.

Composite tissue engineering may offer a solution to the design of complex osseous structures. Isogai et al. designed a combination approach with a copolymer of poly(lactide-co-glycolide) (PLGA) as separate sheets of scaffolds with chondrocytes and tenocytes that were wrapped with bovine periosteum [Isogai et al., 1999]. Twenty weeks after subcutaneous implantation in athymic rats, the resulting structure was comprised of mature articular cartilage with subchondral bone with a tenocapsule, resembling human phalanges with joints.

Menisci

The dense sheet of fibrous tissue in the inter-articular space of the temporomandibular joint is referred to as a meniscus or a disc. Use of the term 'disc' has lead to comparisons of the TMJ structure with the intervertebral disc (IVD). Some similarities in biochemical composition of the outer portion of the IVD and the TMJ meniscus have been noted [Oegema, 1993; Landesberg et al., 1996; Gruber and Hanley, 1998]. Nevertheless, there are more reasons to favor the term TMJ meniscus.

Menisci of the TMJ and the knee are similar to each other in some respects, with both being significantly different from the intervertebral discs. The intervertebral discs are pillows with two morphologically distinct parts: the outer annulus fibrosus is comprised of collagenous laminae and the inner nucleus pulposus is composed of water, proteoglycans, and collagen. There have been some biochemical and cellular analyses of human intervertebral discs and some studies of disc cells in vitro [Hoelscher et al., 2000].

The TMJ meniscus is thinner in its central portion than at the periphery and the posterior, or retrodiscal, tissue is a bilaminar structure containing dense, vascularized and innervated connective tissue. In a classic analysis of fresh cadaveric TMJs, Rees [1954] resolved many of the controversies about meniscal structure and function. The meniscus is not equally thick, but shows 4 transverse zones or bands, having different contents of elastic fibers. Most of the cells appear to be flattened fibrocytes, but there are occasional clusters of round cells with moderately basophilic matrix that are called chondroid cells. There are complex attachments to the joint capsule, to the bones, and to the muscles, with a true insertion to the lateral pterygoid muscle. He demonstrated that the forward excursion of the condylar ridge relative to the temporal bone, which amounts to at least 15 mm, is comprised of two elements. The maximum movement of the mandibular ridge relative to the meniscus is 8 mm and the meniscus moves between 5 and 9 mm relative to the temporal bone, much of this being stretching. The complexities of this structure and its motion must be integrated in prosthesis design [van Loon et al., 2000].

Abnormalities in the relationship between, or positioning of the meniscus and the articular surfaces of the TMJ are classified as internal derangements, in contrast to the extracapsular disorders of the masticatory muscles, or myofascial ailments. Internal derangements are diagnosed by clicking or popping sounds with pain or limitation of function. Roentgenograms will demonstrate degenerative modifications like erosions or bony spurs, while MRI will reveal meniscal morphology and changes in position upon opening of the mouth. Conservative treatments include rest, use of appliances, heat, non-steroidal anti-inflammatory agents, and physical therapy. Arthroscopic procedures are used in both knee and TMJ settings for lavage, to remove debris, to contour irregularities, to reposition tissue, and to repair discontinuities in the vascularized zones.

It is currently viewed that there are inadequate options for the definitive treatment of degenerative, painful TMJ disorders. Experience has been disappointing for surgical repair of the damaged TMJ [Trumpy et al., 1996]. More promising is the use of natural materials. Using a rabbit model, Feinberg et al. [1995] showed that meniscal replacement with either a dermal graft or a collagen sheet resulted in transient cartilaginous hyperplasia of the articular surfaces with normalization by 18 weeks, in contrast to the articular destruction seen without implants. Puelacher et al. [1994] described an engineered construct for TMJ meniscal replacement, but it contained articular chondrocytes and was implanted in subcutaneous sites in immunocompromised mice. It was not unexpected that the construct produced dense cartilage like the donor articular tissue. It may be valuable to test constructs that have been seeded with dermal or other fibroblasts or elastofibrocytes. More information about the nature of normal meniscal cells will be needed. Nevertheless, it is possible that various cell types could adapt to the meniscal microenvironment.

The knee minisci are composed of dense fibrous connective tissue with a vascularized (red) zone and a less vascularized (white) zone, the former one having a greater potential for repair. There has been some clinical success with resorbable collagen meniscus implants followed for 2 years [Rodkey et al., 1999]. Recent work on engineered grafts for knee meniscal repair may lead the way for TMJ meniscal applications. Meniscal repair with a fibrocartilage appearance was achieved in a rabbit partial meniscectomy model in which collagen sponges seeded with bone marrow-derived cells had been used [Walsh et al., 1999]. Empty collagen sponges were also effective in supporting a largely fibrous repair. Untreated lesions did not heal and progressed to degeneration of the joints. Recently, a construct of autogenous, expanded articular chondrocytes that were seeded into a processed allogeneic meniscal segment was used to repair a bucket-handle incision in the avascular zone of the porcine knee meniscus [Peretti et al., 2001]. Scaffold alone or empty incisions did not heal during the 9-week observation period.

More biologic information is needed before progress can be made in engineering the TMJ or its meniscus. There is some information about the characterization of the TMJ meniscal cells [Landesberg et al., 1996], but more needs to be known about the effect of avascularity on meniscal cell differentiation, the potential for avascular tissue repair, and the relationship between meniscal cells and chondrocytes, fibrocytes, and cells of other elastic tissues.

Challenges

Temporomandibular joint disorders that involve internal anatomical defects are approachable by innovative cell-based and cell-free surgical procedures. A major requirement of engineered tissues and organs is that they need to be integrated with the host tissue. Unpredictable union is a problem even with current methods of cartilage and chondrocyte transfer, but may be solved with carriers with adherent properties (e.g. collagen) [Mizuno and Glowacki, 1996] or with biological glues as adjuncts (e.g. fibrin) [Peretti et al., 1998]. Tissue or organ transfers also need to be united with host vasculature and adequately revascularized throughout. This obstacle may be solved by early implantation of engineered constructs before dense bone is formed. This may have to be balanced against the load-bearing requirements in different sites. It may be solved by design of rigid scaffolds with regional paths or signals for angiogenesis.

Another obstacle is the host inflammatory response to foreign material. Many natural polymers are highly biocompatible, but some synthetic materials release particles, hydrogen ions, and other moieties upon resorption or with wear. The major concern is whether resorbable scaffolds would stimulate invasion of inflammatory cells during critical phases of regeneration. Because of the slow in vivo degradation of commonly used polymers, it is unlikely that reactions to the polymer would interfere with the early critical phases of bone formation. On the other hand, nonresorbable scaffolds should be highly biocompatible and not change with time in situ. An implanted construct has to withstand mechanical forces, especially in weight-bearing locations.

Three-dimensional printing or stereolithography has the potential for fabricating complex structures with focal signals. Other approaches being evaluated include scaffold delivery or cell-mediated delivery of angiogenic genes. Cell-free systems with highly engineered biomimetic, or 'smart', materials are intended to modulate the formation of reactive tissues [Healy et al., 1999]. The simplest solution would be to use an off-the-shelf scaffold made of a resorbable material that will have specific signaling factors on its surfaces. Thus, the scaffold could convey important regulatory information to the engineered tissue. Other design elements could control the vascularization of the construct. The implant may contain a single component that triggers the entire cascade of tissue development or multiple, sequentially acting signals for preosteoblasts, osteoblasts, capillaries, articular chondrocytes, and soft tissues, such as synovial, tendon and ligament inserts, discs, or menisci.

Many materials, design approaches, and manufacturing methods are amenable to tissue engineering for repair of bones and joints. It is unlikely that a single approach will solve all problems of tissue and organ regeneration. Within the domain of musculoskeletal tissue and organ engineering, there are likely to be multiple solutions depending upon the particular application.

Acknowledgments

The author's research summarized herein has been supported by NIH grants AR 44873 and AR 455870. Discussions with Drs. Meredith August, David Zaleske, Florin Allemann, and Karen E. Yates are gratefully acknowledged.

References

Allemann, F., S. Mizuno, K. Eid, K.E. Yates, D. Zaleske, J. Glowacki (2001) Effects of hyaluronan on engineered articular cartilage extracellular matrix gene expression in 3-dimensional collagen scaffolds. J Biomed Mater Res *55:* 13–19.

Allemann, F., K.E. Yates, J. Glowacki (2000) Preservation of chondroblastic gene expression signature in 3-D culture devices. J Bone Mineral Res *15:* S468.

Boyan, B.D., C.H. Lohmann, J. Romero, Z. Schwartz (1999) Bone and cartilage tissue engineering. Clin Plast Surg *26:* 629–645.

Boyne P.J., R.E. Marx, M. Nevins, et al. (1997) A feasibility study evaluating rhBMP-2/absorbable collagen sponge for maxillary sinus floor augmentation. Int J Periodont Rest Dent *17:* 11–25.

Brittberg, M., A. Lindhal, A. Nilsson, et al. (1994) Treatment of deep cartilage defects in the knee with autologous chondrocyte transplantation. N Engl J Med *331:* 889–895.

Caruso, E.M., K.U. Lewandrowski, C. Ohlendorf, W.W. Tomford, D. J. Zaleske (1996) Repopulation of laser-perforated chondroepiphyseal matrix with xenogeneic chondrocytes. J Orthop Res *14:* 102–107.

Feinberg, S.E., E. J. McDonnell (1995) The use of a collagen sheet as a disc replacement in the rabbit temporomandibular joint. J Oral Maxillofac Surg *53:* 535–542.

Friedenstein, A.J., I.I. Piatetzky-Shapiro, K.V. Petrakova (1966) Osteogenesis in transplants of bone marrow cells. J Embryol Exp Morphol *16:* 381–390.

Glowacki, J. (2000) In vitro engineering of cartilage. J Rehabil Res Dev *37:* 171–178.
Glowacki, J., S. Mizuno, J.S. Greenberger (1998a) Perfusion enhances functions of bone marrow stromal cells in three-dimensional culture. Cell Trans *7:* 319–326.
Glowacki, J., K. Yates, G. Little, S. Mizuno (1998b) Induced chondroblastic differentiation of human fibroblasts by three-dimensional culture with demineralized bone matrix. Mat Sci Eng C *6:* 199–203.
Goshima, J., V.M. Goldberg, A.I. Caplan (1991) The origin of bone formed in composite grafts of porous calcium phosphate ceramic loaded with marrow cells. Clin Orthop *269:* 274–283.
Grande, D.A., M.I. Pitman, L. Peterson, et al. (1989) The repair of experimentally produced defects in rabbit articular cartilage by autologous chondrocyte transplantation. J Orthop Res *7:* 208–218.
Gruber, H.E., E.N. Hanley, Jr. (1998) Analysis of aging and degeneration of the human intervertebral disc. Comparison of surgical specimens with normal controls. Spine *23:* 751–757.
Healy, K.E., A. Rezania, R.A. Stile (1999) Designing biomaterials to direct biological responses. Ann NY Acad Sci *875:* 24–35.
Hoelscher, G.L., H.E. Gruber, G. Coldham, J.H. Grigsby, E.N. Hanley, Jr. (2000) Effects of very high antibiotic concentrations on human intervertebral disc cell proliferation, viability, and metabolism in vitro. Spine *25:* 1871–1877.
Hollister, S.J., R.A. Levy, T.M. Chu, J.W. Halloran, S. E. Feinberg (2000) An image-based approach for designing and manufacturing craniofacial scaffolds. Int J Oral Maxillofac Surg *29:* 67–71.
Isogai, N., W. Landis, T.H. Kim, et al. (1999) Formation of phalanges and small joints by tissue engineering. J Bone Joint Surg *81A:* 306–316.
Landesberg, R., E. Takeuchi, J.E. Puzas (1996) Cellular, biochemical and molecular characterization of the bovine temporomandibular joint disc. Arch Oral Biol *41:* 761–767.
Lanza, R.P., R. Langer, W.L. Chick (1997) Principles of Tissue Engineering. Austin, R.G. Landes Company/Academic Press.
Mizuno S., J. Glowacki (1996) Chondroinduction of human dermal fibroblasts by demineralized bone in three-dimensional culture. Exp Cell Res *227:* 89–97.
Mizuno S, J. Glowacki (2000) Effects of 2% and 19% oxygen on matrix production by bovine articular chondrocytes in 3-D culture. J Bone Miner Res *15:* S467.
Mizuno S., T. Tateishi, T. Ushida, et al. (1997) Effects of soluble, insoluble, and mechanical factors on bovine chondrocytes in 3-dimensional culture. Trans 43rd Annual Meet, Orthopedic Res Soc, p 537.
Mueller, S.M., J. Glowacki (2000) Construction and regulation of three-dimensional bone tissue in vitro; in Davies, J.E. (ed): Bone Engineering. Toronto, University of Toronto Press, pp 473–487.
Mueller, S.M., L.C. Gerstenfeld, S. Mizuno, J. Glowacki (1999) Medium perfusion enhances osteogenesis by murine osteosarcoma cells in three-dimensional collagen sponges. J Bone Miner Res *14:* 2118–2127.
Oegema, T.R., Jr. (1993) Biochemistry of the intervertebral disc. Clin Sports Med *12:* 419–439.
Peretti, G.M., M.A. Randolph, E.M. Caruso, F. Rossetti, D.J. Zaleske (1998) Bonding of cartilage matrices with cultured chondrocytes: An experimental model. J Orthop Res *16:* 89–95.
Peretti, G.M., T.J. Gill, J.W. Xu, M.A. Randolph, D.J. Zaleske (2001) Cell-based therapy for meniscus healing: A large animal study. Trans 48th Ann Meet, Orthopedic Res Soc.
Puelacher, W.C., J. Wisser, C.A. Vacanti, et al. (1994) Temporomandibular joint disc replacement made by tissue-engineered growth of cartilage. J Oral Maxillofac Surg *52:* 1172–1177.
Rodkey W.G., J.R. Steadman, S.T. Li (1999) A clinical study of collagen meniscus implants to restore the injured meniscus. Clin Orthop Rel Res *367:* S281–S292.
Ratner B.D., A.S. Hoffman, F.J. Schoen, J.E. Lemons (1996) Biomaterials Science: An Introduction to Materials in Medicine. San Diego, Academic Press.
Rees, L.A. (1954) The structure and function of the mandibular joint. Br Dent J *96:* 125–133.
Sindelar, B.J., S.P. Evanko, T. Alonzo, S.W. Herring, T. Wight (2000) Effects of intraoral splint wear on proteoglycans in the temporomandibular joint disc. Arch Biochem Biophys *379:* 64–70.
Symes, J.F., D.W. Losordo, P.R. Vale, et al. (1999) Gene therapy with vascular endothelial growth factor for inoperable coronary artery disease. Ann Thorac Surg *68:* 830–836.
Temenoff J.S., A. G. Mikos (2000) Review: Tissue engineering for regeneration of articular cartilage. Biomaterials *21:* 431–440.
Trumpy, I.G., B. Roald, T. Lyberg (1996) Morphologic and immunohistochemical observation of explanted Proplast-Teflon temporomandibular joint interpositional implants. J Oral Maxillofac Surg *54:* 63–68.
Vacanti, C.A., R. Langer, B. Schloo, et al. (1991) Synthetic piolymers seeded with chondrocytes provide a template for new cartilage formation. Plast Reconstr Surg *87:* 753–759.
van Loon, J.P., G.J. Verkerke, M.P. de Vries L.G. de Bont (2000) Design and wear testing of a temporomandibular joint prosthesis articulation. J Dent Res *79:* 715–721.
Wakitani, S., T. Goto, S.J. Pineda, et al. (1994) Mesenchymal cell-based repair of large, full-thickness defects of articular cartilage. J Bone Joint Surg Am *76:* 579–592.
Walsh, C.J., D. Goodman, A.I. Caplan, V.M. Goldberg (1999) Meniscus regeneration in a rabbit partial meniscectomy model. Tissue Eng *5:* 327–337.
Zaleske, D.J., S. Kim, E.M. Caruso, G. M. Peretti, K.T. Schomacker, J. Glowacki (1999) Enzymatic pre-treatment of devitalized chick embryonic cartilage matrix for enhancement of seeding/penetration with xenogeneic chondrocytes. Trans 46th Ann Meet, Orthopedic Res Soc, p 684.

Cells
Tissues
Organs

Cells Tissues Organs 2001;169:309–321

Image-Based Biomimetic Approach to Reconstruction of the Temporomandibular Joint

Stephen E. Feinberg[a] Scott J. Hollister[b] John W. Halloran[c]
T.M. Gabe Chu[d] Paul H. Krebsbach[e]

[a]Department of Oral and Maxillofacial Surgery, Schools of Dentistry and Medicine;
[b]Departments of Biomedical Engineering and Mechanical Engineering and Applied Mechanics,
College of Engineering, and Department of Surgery, School of Medicine; [c]Department of Material Sciences and Engineering, College of Engineering; [d]Department of Material Sciences and Engineering, College of Engineering, and School of Dentistry, and [e]Department of Oral Medicine, Pathology and Oncology, School of Dentistry,
University of Michigan, Ann Arbor, Mich., USA

Key Words
Imaged-based · Biomimetic · Reconstruction · Temporomandibular joint

Abstract
This article will present an image-based approach to the designing and manufacturing of biomimetic tissue engineered temporomandibular (TMJ) condylar prosthesis. Our vision of a tissue-engineered TMJ prosthesis utilizes a 3-D designed and manufactured biodegradable scaffold shaped similar to a condylar head and neck, i.e. a condylar-ramus unit (CRU). The fabricated CRU scaffold can be constructed with a specific intra-architectural design such that it will enhance the formation of tissue from implanted cells placed within its interstices. These biologic cues could influence scaffold-implanted mesenchymal stem cells (MSC) or bone marrow stromal cells (BMSC) to form a fibrocartilaginous joint surface, or cap, on top of a bony strut, similar to a costochondral rib graft (CCRG), which could be fixed to the mandibular ramus.

Supported in part by a Research Support Grant award from the Oral and Maxillofacial Surgery Foundation.

Abbreviations used in this paper

BFGF	basic fibroblast growth factor
BMP	bone morphogenetic protein
BMSC	bone marrow stromal cells
CAD	computer-aided design
CCRG	costochondral rib graft
CRU	condylar-ramus unit
CT	computer tomography
3-D	three-dimensional
ECM	extracellular matrix
FDA	Federal Drug Administration
HA	hydroxyapatite
IBE	image-based engineering
LM	layered manufacturing
MRI	magnetic resonance imaging
MSC	mesenchymal stem cells
PDGF	platelet-derived growth factor
PGA	polyglycolic acid
PLA	polylactide acid
PTFE	polytetrafluroethylene
RP	rapid prototyping
SFF	solid free-form fabrication
SL	stereolithography
TCP	tricalcium phosphate
TGF-β	transforming growth factor beta
TMJ	temporomandibular joint
UV	ultraviolet

KARGER
Fax +41 61 306 12 34
E-Mail karger@karger.ch
www.karger.com

1422–6405/01/1693–0309$17.50/0

Accessible online at:
www.karger.com/journals/cto

Dr. Stephen E. Feinberg
Department of Oral and Maxillofacial Surgery
B1-B204 UH, Box 0018
1500 E Medical Center Dr., Ann Arbor, MI 48109-0018 (USA)
Tel. +1 734 763 5963, Fax +1 734 936 5941, E-Mail sefein@umich.edu

This new approach to tissue engineering a TMJ would be advantageous because of its patient site-specific anatomical configuration as well as its potential ability to adapt to the loading forces placed on it during function.

Introduction

One of the major obstacles that have plagued the reconstruction of the temporomandibular joint (TMJ) has been the adverse reaction seen with the use of alloplastic, nonbiologic materials. These inert and passive materials, by themselves, do not respond to normal biochemical or mechanical biologic signals which are present in situ within the TMJ. The patient, because of the biological inertness of these materials, must adapt to the material or mechanical device that has been used. This usually results in associated problems with a compromised functional outcome [Rubin et al., 1997]. At present there is only one Federal Drug Administration (FDA) approved synthetic total joint replacement for the TMJ. This is manufactured by TMJ Concepts, Inc. [Sampson et al., 1999]. TMJ Concepts basic approach is similar to that of ours in the use of imaging a site-specific area to be reconstructed, TMJ, and then to manufacture the prosthesis off of the image dataset for each patient. The main difference between our two approaches is that ours uses biological interactive and viable tissue elements versus their use of noninteractive alloplastic materials.

The use of viable autogenous tissue offers an exciting alternative to the options of alloplasts and nonbiologic materials. Autogenous tissue has an advantage of the ability to respond to biologic cues but has the disadvantages of donor site morbidity, limitation of quantity of available tissue and an acceptance of less than perfect anatomic match for the tissue being replaced or reconstructed. Previous alloplastic devices have been unsuccessful in the past because patients must adapt to the implanted synthetic, nonviable TMJ prosthesis [Mercuri, 1998; Van Loon et al., 1995]. In contrast, the use of autogenous tissue for total TMJ repair or reconstruction, allows biological remodeling of the implant to occur by the functional forces placed on it by the patient. This, in fact, may be the major reason the use of costochondral rib grafts (CCRG) for TMJ reconstruction has been so successful.

The successful use of autogenous CCRGs has been attributed to the presence of a cartilaginous cap atop of the bony strut of the rib [Perrot et al., 1994; Raustia et al., 1996]. Studies have shown that condylar cartilage, associated with the fibrocartilaginous articular surface, enables the TMJ to withstand compression and loading which assists in the morphological adaptive responses to biomechanical stress [Meikle, 1992]. In addition, it has been shown that mechanical stimuli elicited by joint function can determine the ultimate growth and shape of the condyle [Copray et al., 1985]. However, the CCRG has the disadvantages of both donor site morbidity and being poorly shaped for anatomical placement within the TMJ region.

The development and use of biologically responsive materials will allow modulation, in situ, of the grafted or reconstructed tissue so that it addresses the unique needs and demands of that specific anatomic site and/or function. A tissue engineering/biomimetic approach may allow us to develop a new prosthesis that could eliminate or minimize the disadvantages of the use of biological tissues, donor site morbidity and poor anatomical shape, but yet take advantage of its positive attributes, adaptively to functional forces.

Our vision of a tissue-engineered TMJ prosthesis utilizes a 3-D designed and manufactured biodegradable scaffold shaped similar to a condylar head and neck, i.e. a condylar-ramus unit (CRU) (fig. 1). The fabricated CRU scaffold would be constructed such that it will have, at the time of placement, the mechanical structure to withstand the functional forces of joint loading imparted upon it. In addition, the intra-architectural design would be fabricated in such a way, i.e. pore size, channel orientation, etc., as to maximize vascular and tissue ingrowth into the scaffold. The scaffold could be made 'smart' by incorporation of specific types of collagen and/or growth factors to impart biologic cues to scaffold-implanted mesenchymal stem cells (MSC) or bone marrow stromal cells (BMSC) to 'push' them to form a fibrocartilaginous joint surface, or cap, on top of a bony strut, similar to a costochondral rib graft (CCRG), which could then be fixated to the mandibular ramus. This new approach to tissue engineering a TMJ would be advantageous because of its site-specific anatomical configuration as well as its potential ability to adapt to the loading forces placed on it during function.

Principles of Tissue Engineering and Biomimetics

Within the last decade the newly emerging field of tissue engineering has developed to a level of sophistication that it now may offer alternatives for TMJ reconstruction. Tissue engineering is defined as the application of principles of biomimetics for the restoration, repair, replace-

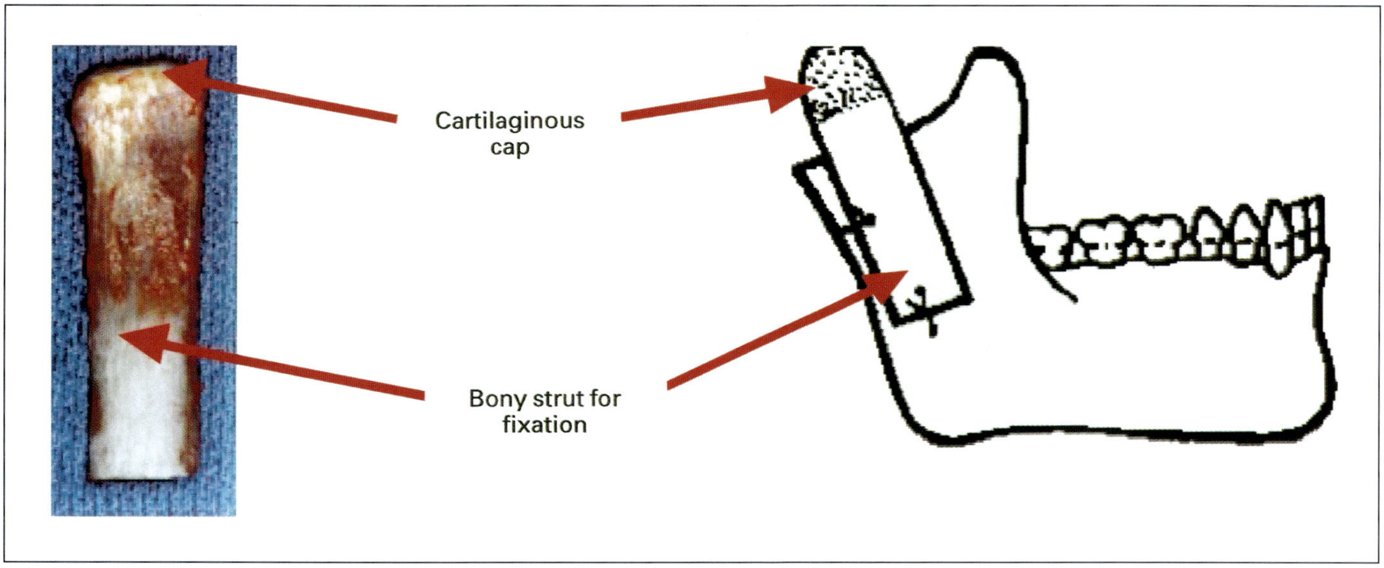

Fig. 1. Illustration of a costochondral rib graft, on the left, placed, schematically, on the right, on the ramus of the mandible, in a standard surgical approach in the reconstruction of the TMJ.

ment and assembly of functional tissue and organs [Langer and Vacanti, 1993]. Biomimetics is defined as an interdisciplinary field that combines information from the study of biological structures and their function with physics, mathematics, chemistry and engineering in the development of principles that are important for the generation of novel synthetic materials and organs.

In the past, reconstructive joint surgery focused on the designing of replacement parts for the TMJ. With the debut of tissue engineering and biomimetics the focus has shifted to reconstruction using functional biological components of tissues. The ex vivo construction of a TMJ replacement, using a biomimetic approach, will involve several components: (1) stem cells or progenitor populations; (2) regulatory signals such as growth factors or mechanotransductional forces, and (3) biodegradable and compatible scaffolds with specific architecture to include the extracellular matrix and/or the suprastructure (external and internal) of the reconstructive region.

These three components must follow the cardinal rules of tissue engineering. First, optimal regulatory signals must be present, second, the cells must be able to respond to these regulatory signals, and third, one must have an instructive and interactive scaffold whose geometry and surface coating can influence cells that migrate in and/or attach to it.

In this article we will focus on the instructive and interactive scaffold component of tissue engineering. Specifically, we outline and demonstrate an image-based method to design and manufacture 3-dimensional (3-D) scaffolds for TMJ reconstruction.

Scaffolds

A scaffold can be defined as a transitional physiochemical framework within which cells populating it create a replacement tissue as the prosthesis disappears or is incorporated into the surrounding tissues. The optimal properties for fabrication of scaffolds from biomaterials have been outlined by Bell [1995]. The ideal scaffold should be biodegradable and nontoxic, have degradation products that are nontoxic, should allow cell attachment, and should be able to be remodeled by the cells. The physical properties of the scaffold should be similar to those of the tissue it is replacing with respect to strength, compliance, and density. The scaffold should be a good substrate for the extracellular matrix (ECM) enzymes to modify it as necessary. The scaffold should also allow cell motility and ingress of angiogenic elements while having a low level of immunogenicity and thrombogenicity and should be capable of being fixated, if necessary, with screws or sutures. Finally, the scaffold must be interactive with its surrounding environment.

The different types of scaffolds that are available fall into three basic categories: (1) Non-bioabsorbable (manmade materials with little or no information content for cells, i.e. Dacron, nylon, polytetrafluroethylene [PTFE]). (2) Bioabsorbable (manmade with low information content for cells, i.e. polylactic acid [PLA], polyglycolic acid [PGA]; combinations of PLA/PGA, and calcium phosphates ceramics [hydroxyapatite {HA}, tricalcium phosphates {TCP}]). (3) Naturally occurring materials with high information content for cells (secreted biomatrix, animal and human tissues [dermis, dura, ligaments, heart valves]; or animal polymers [collagens, elastin, laminins, fibronectin, glycosaminoglycans]).

Role of Interactive Scaffolds

Scaffolds should be enriched with instructive materials that could be interactive and influence host and/or seeded cell production of the ECM. It is only through this approach that we will be able to accurately fabricate functional tissue replacement parts [Bell, 1995]. This could be accomplished by making the scaffolds responsive to site-specific needs of the area to be reconstructed, i.e. TMJ. One way to accomplish this is by controlling the degradation rate of the scaffold such that it is replaced seamlessly by natural tissue. Another alternative approach is to control the surface properties of the scaffold such that this could influence or determine the types of cells that attach to the scaffold, their behavior, growth, differentiation and/or migration through the scaffold. One could also control the 3-D internal architectural structure, such as pore size, channel direction and trabecular orientation, as well as surface chemistry or local surface texture of the scaffold as is seen on dental implant surfaces.

What is most important about this approach to reconstructive surgery is the ability to create a dynamic functional interaction between the cells and the scaffold. This is seen when cells synthesize and secrete multiple molecules into the surrounding immediate environment to form an ECM. The secreted ECM can impart important signals and properties to the scaffold. Collagen fibrils secreted within the ECM can enhance tensile strength, whereas release of proteoglycans, or ground substances, that are incorporated into the ECM can bind fluid to improve the compressive properties as is seen in cartilage. The secretion of cytokines or growth factors into the surrounding environment can influence cell growth and behavior (BMP, PDGF, bFGF, TGF-β). Specific cell surface receptors can interact with the ECM and scaffold affecting cell behavior, attachment, migration and/or differentiation.

The signal transmission between cells and the ECM can be accomplished through several means, one of which is mechanotransduction. This is germane to reconstruction of a TMJ since it is considered a loaded joint under force. The signal could be either a solid deformation resulting directly from muscle and bite forces or a fluid flow effect secondary to deformation. The importance of an interactive 3-D scaffold coated with an ECM is illustrated in a study in which hepatocytes are placed into two different environments. One is a nonphysiologic environment in which the ECM or collagen is in contact with the cells only on one side (not naturally seen in vivo). The second is a more natural environment in which the hepatocytes are placed in contact with collagen (ECM) on both sides (a situation more typical in the liver). If one compares cell function of the hepatocytes, as measured by their secretion of bile salts, protein and urea, the cells in the more natural environment, collagen on both sides, will secrete exponentially more of these products [Dunn et al., 1991].

Mechanotransduction can influence cell and scaffold interactions through stretch-activated stress channels through ECM connections within the cytoskeleton via integrins [Ingber, 1993] such that mechanical loading could influence matrix synthesis assembly and degradation. This is illustrated by the work of Guldberg [1997] and others in a pneumatically loaded bone chamber which was placed into the tibial plateau of canines. The forces in the chamber were then varied and assessed for bone formation. The chambers that were mechanically loaded showed a higher density of bone formation than the unloaded chambers.

In summary, in order to obtain an optimal reconstructive outcome one would need to control all of the variables; cells, growth factors, scaffold makeup and design, as well as the interactions between all of the above. The ability to control or direct these variables would enable successful site-specific anatomical reconstruction.

Importance of Intra-Architectural Scaffold Geometry

A scaffold for a TMJ prosthesis should provide interactive and/or functional biologic cues or signals to guide incremental matrix production by either invading or implanted cells [Bell, 1995]. The architectural design of the scaffold/matrix should also be instrumental in influencing biological activity (cell infiltration, attachment, differentiation and function) and mechanical integrity (ability to withstand or distribute mechanical forces) [Ingber, 1993].

Several studies have shown that scaffold pore size can influence formation of bone or cartilage regeneration. Coralline HA scaffolds, with a pore size of 500 μm, allowed extensive cellular and vascular invasion and new bone formation after 12 weeks in vivo, while no bone formation or cellular invasion was found within 200-μm scaffolds [Kuhne et al., 1994]. Gauthier and others [1998], utilizing macroporous biphasic calcium phosphate ceramics, showed a 563-μm pore size provided more new bone formation, both in peripheral and deep pores, than a 300-μm pore size. Tsuruga et al. [1997] noted that a HA structure with pore sizes of 300–400 μm, complexed with rhBMP-2, was optimal for attachment, differentiation and growth of osteoblasts and for vascular ingrowth. Kuboki et al. [1995] showed that rhBMP induced only osteogenesis when porous particles of HA were used as a carrier, whereas only chondrogenesis occurred within a carrier of fibrous glass membrane. They concluded that vasculature was the crucial factor that determined osteogenesis or chondrogenesis. The findings of Tsuruga et al. [1997] and Kuboki et al. [1995] showed that scaffold geometry, which restricted vascular invasion, would produce cartilage while other geometries that could accommodate a haversian system, would produce bone. Jin et al. [2000] showed that BMP-induced bone formation is highly dependent on the geometry of the carrier, which provides feasible structure factors for vascularization. Ripamonti and Reddi [1992] showed that pore sizes of 150 μm could not support neovascularization. These studies demonstrate the significant effect scaffold pore size can have on bone or cartilage regeneration and vascular ingrowth.

The use of pluripotent cells on HA ceramic scaffolds is a promising approach for the engineering of a hard tissue construct. HA scaffolds, though, because of their brittleness will most likely not be beneficial in loaded areas as the TMJ. Either mesenchymal stem cells (MSC) or bone marrow stem cells (BMSC) can regenerate bone and, if given the appropriate microenvironment, may also regenerate cartilage. Bruder et al. [1998] and Dennis et al. [1992] noted bone formation in a rat femoral defect model when a porous ceramic carrier was loaded with MSCs. Negligible bone formation was noted in carriers without MSCs. Kadiyala et al. [1997] saw both bone and cartilage formation in porous ceramic carriers loaded with canine MSCs implanted subcutaneously into dogs and mice. Krebsbach et al. [1997, 1999] found significant bone formation in mice with HA/TCP carriers loaded with BMSCs. These results indicate that cells from marrow

User selects defect region for reconstruction from CT/MRI

↓

Define the tissue replacement area by image processing and digitization (*external* scaffold design)

↓

Design and optimize site-specific *internal* architecture within the external scaffold design

↓

Create the .stl or similar format from image data to direct a layer manufacturing machine; an approach denoted as solid free-form fabrication (SFF)

↓

Scaffold Image surface extracted to create .stl data

↓

Impart instructive or functional biological elements within or on the scaffold

Fig. 2. Basic steps involved in designing an instructive scaffold for TMJ reconstruction.

stroma have the capacity to form significant amounts of bone and/or cartilage when placed in defects with either HA or HA/TCP ceramic scaffolds.

In summary, stromal cells have the potential to regenerate bone and/or cartilage when placed on bioceramic scaffolds. The geometry or pore size of a biomaterial scaffold carrier can play an important role in the type and amount of tissue regenerated. The recent advances in biomaterial stereolithography [Brady et al., 1996] and image-based design methods [Hollister et al., 1997], allow us to study the effect of scaffold architecture (pore size) on bone and cartilage regeneration of bioceramic scaffolds loaded with marrow stromal cells [Krebsbach et al., 1997, 1999]. Finally, these techniques will have to be adapted to new biomaterials that can be placed into areas that will be loaded, such as the TMJ. This will most likely be done with a new generation of self-reinforced biodegradable polymers.

An Image-Based Approach to Design and Manufacture of a TMJ Condylar-Ramus Unit Construct

Our image-based approach to the design and manufacture of a condylar-ramus unit (CRU) scaffold for TMJ reconstruction consists of 5 basic steps (fig. 2).

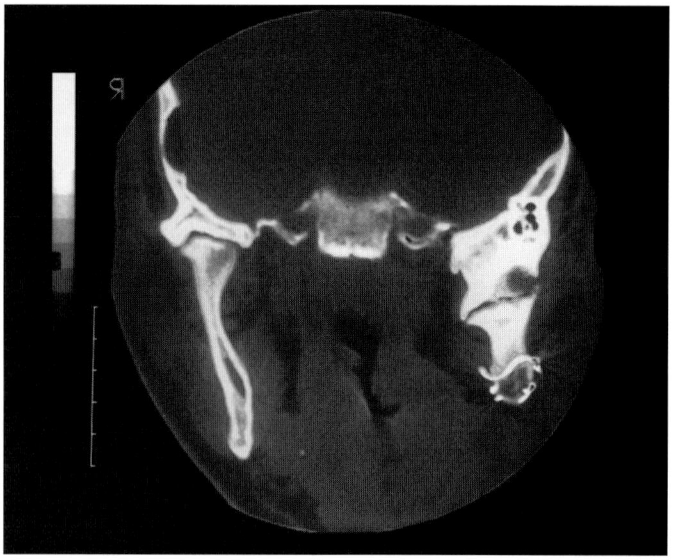

Fig. 3. Coronal CT cut showing a normal TMJ on the right side and a severely degenerated and deformed TMJ on the left side. The mirror image of the normal right side could be used as a template for a scaffold to reconstruct the abnormal left side.

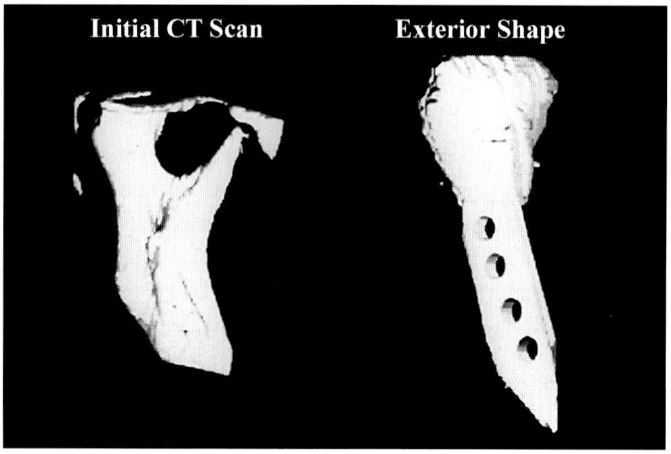

Fig. 4. Step 1: External scaffold shape and definition. View of external scaffold shape constructed from CT data. Left: 3-D image of CT data. Right: General 3-D view of external scaffold shape.

(1) Assess and image the TMJ to be reconstructed by magnetic resonance imaging (MRI) and/or computer tomography (CT).

(2) Define the tissue replacement area by image processing and digitization (the external scaffold design).

(3) Design and optimize site-specific internal architecture within the external scaffold design.

(4) Create the stl. or similar format from image data to direct a layered manufacturing machine; an approach denoted as solid free-form fabrication (SFF).

(5) Impart instructive or functional biological elements within or on the scaffold.

Step 1: Assess and Image the TMJ to Be Reconstructed by MRI and/or CT

In a majority of elective maxillofacial procedures, especially in TMJ reconstruction, imaging of the area to be reconstructed with a CT and/or MRI scan is routinely done (fig. 3, 4).

In the last several years our team at the University of Michigan [Hollister et al., 1997; Zysset, 1997; Hollister et al., 1998, 2000] has developed an approach to designing anatomic structures using image datasets. This method, denoted here as image-based engineering (IBE), allows rapid construction of complex 3-D (3-D) geometry. A particular advantage for reconstruction of the TMJ is that IBE techniques can be readily coupled with common clinical imaging modalities like CT and MRI to create patient/anatomic specific biomaterial scaffolds. In addition, one can create complex porous architectures and then combine it with the exterior anatomy using Boolean image processing operations [Hollister et al., 1998]. This allows one to rigorously control the internal architecture of biomaterial scaffolds to include pore size, geometry and orientation.

Step 2: Define the Tissue Replacement Area by Image Processing and Digitization (External Scaffold Design)

A commercial software program such as PV-Wave (Visual Numerics, Inc., Boulder, Colo., USA) or IDL (Interactive Data Language, Research Systems, Inc., Boulder, Colo., USA) is used to read the CT or MRI data of the image of the TMJ region to be reconstructed. The external geometry of the defect area is outlined and then by inverting the contrast of the image a 3-D image of the defect or area to be reconstructed can be generated (fig. 5). The image of the reconstruction area specifies the contour design of the scaffold necessary for reconstruction of the area in concert with the surrounding adjacent tissue. This user interactive process creates a second set of data for the design methodology, which is denoted as the 'defect image'. The advantage of this approach is the speed and ease in which complicated scaffold designs can be constructed.

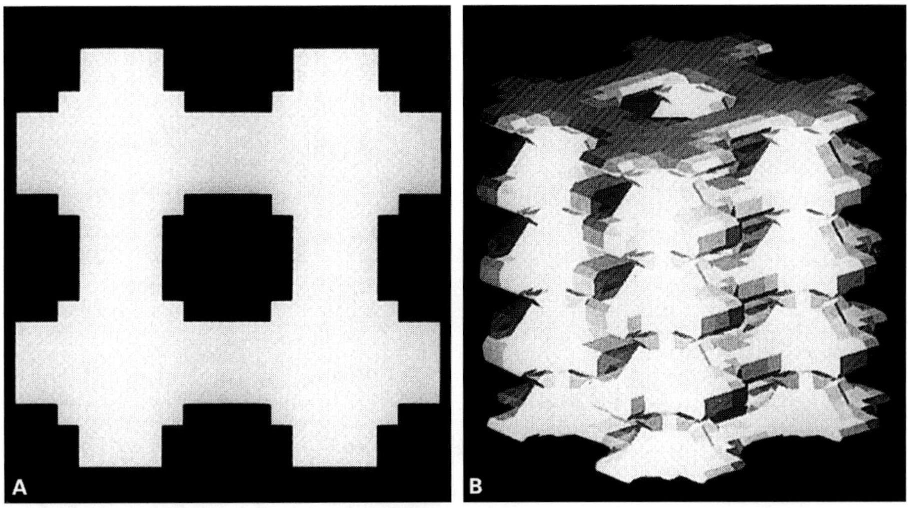

Fig. 5. Step 2: Internal scaffold architecture. Internal ellipsoid shaped porous internal architecture with pore diameter of 700 μm. Repeating a basic unit cell creates the porous architecture. **A** Slice through image of one unit cell. Solid material is white. **B** 3-D surface rendering of a collection of the unit cells that create the internal architecture.

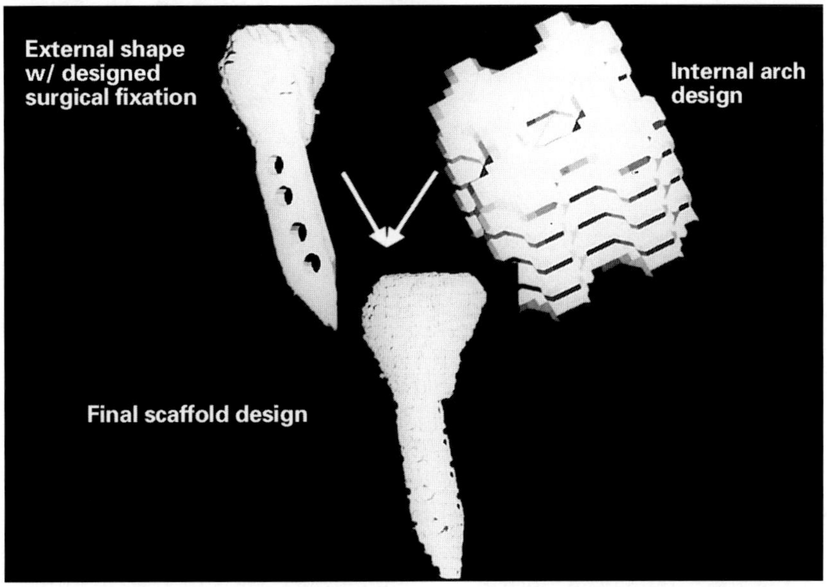

Fig. 6. Step 3: Synthesized scaffold design by Boolean operations by combining step 1, the external scaffold design, with step 2, the internal scaffold architecture.

Step 3: Design and Optimize Site-Specific Internal Architecture within the External Scaffold Design

In this step, we define the internal scaffold architecture. The internal architectural design is composed of pore size, channel size and orientation, etc. This could be determined empirically or patterned from the normal or native architectural design of the area to be reconstructed. This is easily done especially if the contralateral TMJ is intact and thus could be used as a template (fig. 3).

The first step in scaffold design is to create the internal pore architecture. The internal pore architecture will determine crucial factors for tissue regeneration including nutrient diffusion, cell and tissue infiltration and mechanical behavior. Although internal architecture must be selected carefully since it can greatly influence matrix deposition, optimizing internal architecture will require extensive in vitro and in vivo experiments. A wide variety of experimental designs are necessary as input to experimentation for determining the optimal parameters.

The idea behind image-based topology design is simply to set voxels, which are 3-D pixels, within an image design cube to either 0 for no material or 1 for material. The basic cube is repeated as many times as possible to create the architecture image. A general program is created to construct an internal architecture by repeating a unit structure. Using geometric mathematical formulas, images can

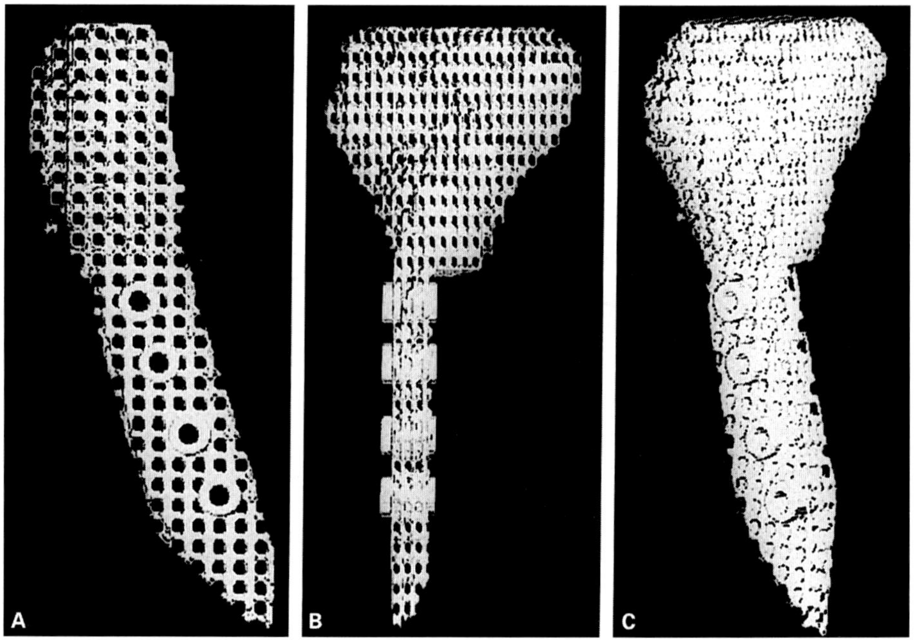

Fig. 7. Final instructive scaffold by Boolean combination of external scaffold design with internal scaffold design with internal scaffold architecture manufactured from a stl. file. **A** Sagittal view showing porous scaffold with sleeves designed to incorporate fixation screws. **B** Coronal view of the same scaffold with fixation sleeves. **C** General 3-D view of the completed instructive scaffold.

be created of cylinders, spheres and other similar entities. With this approach, interior architectural channels can be created to allow for cell infiltration and tissue ingrowth (fig. 6).

The above method creates a regular pore structure. Image-based topology design can also be used to create random porous structures. One way is to run randomly set voxels to 0 or 1 using a random number generator. A second method to create pores is by adjusting thresholds of the original defect image [Hollister et al., 1998]. By setting all voxel densities outside a narrow threshold range to zero, all of the trabecular bone and also random pores within the cortical bone are created. Using this technique, the pore size will be determined by the image resolution as mm/voxel.

Steps 2 and 3 produce two separate datasets: (1) the defect image (external geometry) which is the anatomic location where the structure will be placed, and (2) the architecture image, which is an image of the internal architectural pore structure. At this point, using image processing software and setting the solid and void voxel densities in the defect image, the interior architecture image and void spaces to different values, we can combine the defect image with the architecture image. This is done by assigning the void space in both images a density of 0, the solid portions of the defect image a density of 250, and the solid portions of the architecture image a density of 200. These different densities allow us to use Boolean operations to combine the pixel values. It is also possible in this step to incorporate specific design characteristics into the scaffold, such as, differential internal geometric cues that could induce bone versus cartilage, or incorporation of a tidemark to separate bone from cartilage as well as 'sleeves' or 'female' internal structures to assist in fixation (fig. 6, 7).

Once the external scaffold shape and internal scaffold architecture are defined via Boolean operations, they can be converted into a 3-D finite element model to simulate in vivo loading. An image-based finite element modeling and fully stressed topology optimization software (Voxelcon, Voxel Computing, Inc., Ann Arbor, Mich., USA) can be used to preduct strategic locations to increase bone mass in 3-D constructs to reduce stress that might initiate failure in the scaffold (fig. 8).

This step can be used to further modify 3-D scaffold designs to reduce stress, which might initiate failure of the scaffold in vivo. In essence, we can predict mechanical performance of the site-specific designed scaffold before implantation. If the scaffold is biodegradable, then one has to take into consideration the degradation of the scaffold in unison with tissue infiltration and deposition such that the mechanical performance of the scaffold is maintained. Once this is complete, a stl. file can be made to computer-generate the final configuration and shape of the scaffold (fig. 7).

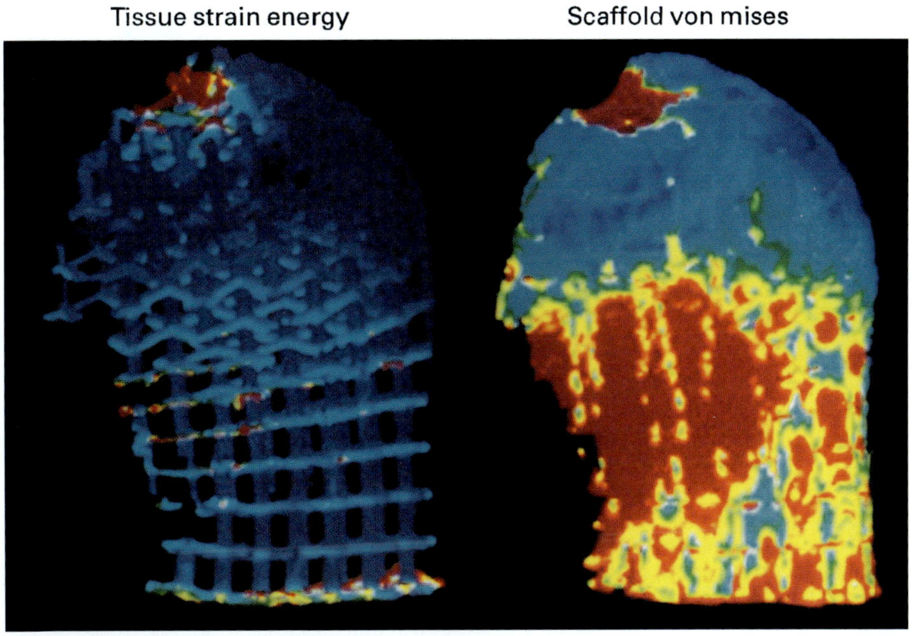

Fig. 8. Stress analysis of scaffold simulated with tissue ingrowth. Left: Picture shows strain energy in ingrown tissue. Right: Von Mises stress in scaffold.

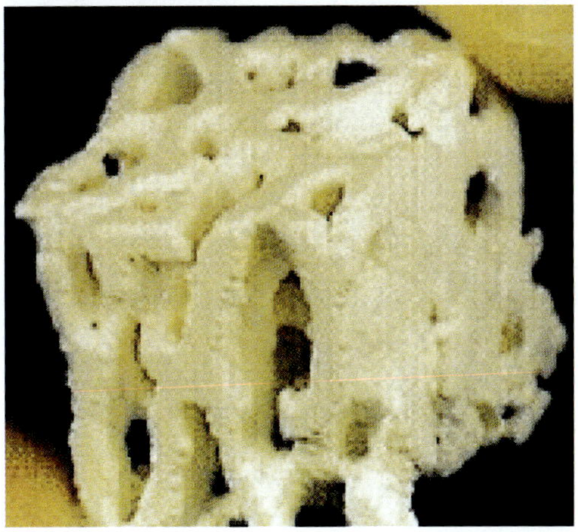

Fig. 9. A 2-mm cube of a human distal femoral trabecular bone manufactured from alumina oxide on a stereolithography machine. This gives an example of the complex 3-D architectures that may be built into instructive scaffolds.

In summary, the literature seems to indicate that intra-architectural design can influence diffusion pathways of nutrients, mechanical compliance, and mechanotransductive forces on the invading tissue or implanted cells.

Step 4: Create an Image Format to Direct a Machine to Manufacture the Scaffold via a Solid Free-Form Fabrication (SFF) Technique

Once the digital image representation of the external and internal scaffold design is completed, the scaffold can be manufactured using solid free-form fabrication (SFF) techniques. SFF refers to a set of techniques developed in the past decade for directly building solid physical objects from computer files. SFF techniques are used to create plastic engineering models from computer-aided design (CAD) files, or to create plastic anatomical models from medical CT files. A solid object, with a complex shape, is produced from a sequence of many thin slices, so the process is often called layered manufacturing (LM). The most important commercial application of SFF is the rapid production of engineering prototypes, or rapid prototyping (RP).

Creating external shape has been the goal for SFF, but these techniques can also be used to create an internal architecture. This makes SFF an ideal method to manu-

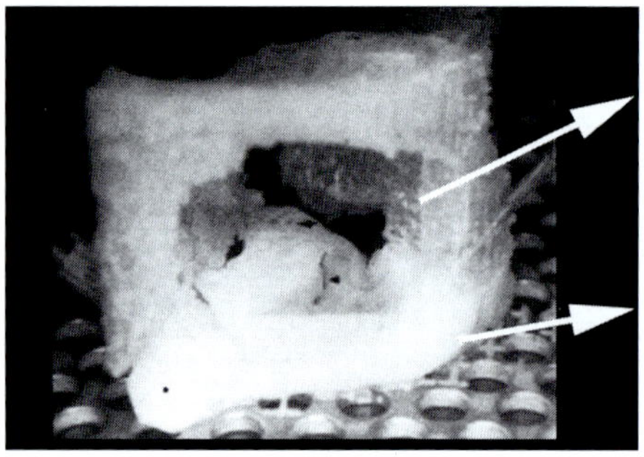

10

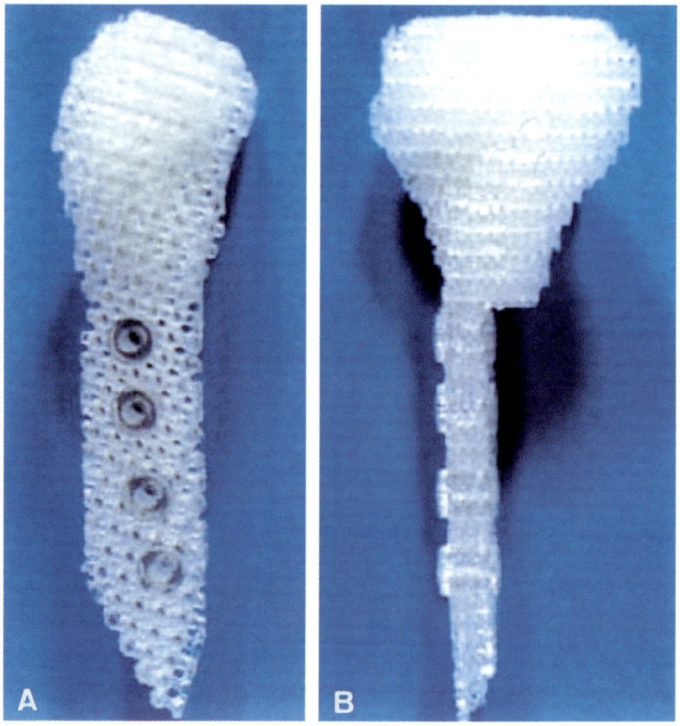

11

Fig. 10. A hydroxyapatite orbital floor scaffold that was designed and manufactured per our protocol off of a human skull.

Fig. 11. Final scaffold of a condylar-ramus unit made of polyurethane manufactured from a stl. file on a stereolithographic machine. **A** Sagittal view. **B** Coronal view. Observe that sleeves have been placed for fixation screws as well as the porous nature of the scaffold. Compare with figure 7.

facture implant microstructures with a precisely designed architecture. In order to achieve this for HA or polymer biomaterial implants, however, we must have SFF techniques, which are capable of achieving pore sizes down to 150 μm and are applicable to fabrication from implantable biomaterials. The Advanced Ceramics Laboratory at the University of Michigan has recently developed a process for SFF of hydroxyapatite (HA) ceramics using stereolithography (SL).

Stereolithography is a process that creates solid objects layer-by-layer, using a computer-driven ultraviolet (UV) laser to photopolymerize layers of liquid resin [Jacobs, 1992]. After each layer is cured, a fresh layer of liquid resin is applied, and the next solid layer is photopolymerized. The process is repeated for several thousand layers over the course of several hours, leading to solid plastic models of remarkable detail and accuracy. An alumina oxide model of human trabecular tissue was created from a micro-CT file, built at 8 times life size (fig. 9) [Zysset et al., 1997]. This demonstrated the ability to create a complex object with detailed interconnecting solid and void phase. The file to create this part had 626,000 facets in the STL file.

We have adapted the SL process to build ceramics using a fluid suspension of ceramic powder in a photopolymerizable acrylate liquid [Griffith et al., 1995]. The ceramic objects are built layer-by-layer in a commercial stereolithography apparatus (SLA250/40, 3D Systems, Inc., Valencia, Calif., USA), with the photocured acrylate serving as a 'binder' to hold together the fine ceramic powders. After the 'build' is completed, the ceramic + acrylate solid is heated to 500°C to remove the acrylate, and is subsequently fired at high temperature (1,200–1,600°C) to sinter the ceramic. Chu et al. [1997, 1998] has developed a fluid suspension of HA ceramic powder that can be used either directly in the SLA250 apparatus or indirectly by casting the suspension into epoxy models built on SLA250. The cured suspension is subsequently sintered to a dense HA ceramic. We have used this technique to successfully construct an orbit floor HA scaffold (fig. 10) [Levy et al., 1997].

To be able to produce a ceramic scaffold with a specific internal and external geometry, it is necessary to represent the structure (scaffold) in a data format known a stereolithography or stl., which defines the surface(s) as connected triangles. Therefore, in previous step 2, an isosurface density is extracted to produce a triangular facet representation of the surface (Voxelcon 2.0, Voxel Computing, Inc., Ann Arbor, Mich., USA). This process is automated and produces an ASCII text file with vertices and normals of the triangular facets that will be able to run the stereolithographic machine. We have been successful in using this approach to manufacture a TMJ CRU construct from polyurethane as a demonstration of the efficacy of this technique (fig. 11).

The ultimate goal is to adapt the use of solid free-form fabrication manufacturing to the use of either a biodegradable polymer or in combination with a calcium phosphate ceramic since HA is too brittle to place in a load-bearing area by itself. Studies in our laboratory are presently ongoing to develop this approach with an FDA-approved self-reinforced biodegradable polymer in conjunction with various SFF manufacturing techniques.

Step 5: Impart Instructive or Functional Biological Elements within or on the Scaffold

The ultimate goal of our biomimetic approach to reconstruction of the TMJ by fabrication of a condylar-ramus unit (CRU) construct is the formation of cartilage and bone on the same scaffold. One means to accomplishing this goal is by making site-specific interactive scaffolds. In an effort to make scaffolds more instructive or interactive several approaches can be undertaken. First, one can add either growth factors and/or various extracellular matrix proteins that are capable of regulating cell attachment, migration, proliferation, and differentiation. These proteins can impart an inductive component by providing chemical cues to initiate and maintain the processes of bone and/or cartilage formation at site-specific areas within the scaffold(s). This was shown to be successfully accomplished with the use of type I or II collagens which were able to impart biological cues to MSCs to differentiate into either osteoblasts or chondrocytes, respectively, to form bone or cartilage [Shi et al., 1996; Kadiyala et al., 1997; Nehrer et al., 1997].

Others have shown that specific cytokines or growth factors, such as transforming growth factor-β1 (TGF-β) and/or basic fibroblast growth factor (bFGF) can stimulate chondrogenesis and inhibit osteogenesis [Iwasaki et al., 1993, 1995; Izumi et al., 1992]. Others have shown that different growth factors, such as bone morphogenetic protein (BMP), may play a prominent role in formation of bone [Brekke and Toth, 1998].

Incorporation of an osteogenic plasmid gene into the scaffold is another novel approach to induce bone formation. In this approach plasmid DNA containing bone morphogenetic protein-4 and/or parathyroid hormone is incorporated within degradable collagen matrices and placed into a segmental gap defect in an adult rat femur. The invading fibroblasts, the first cells to enter for repair of the defect, were able to 'take up' the expression plasmid DNA resulting in faster formation of new bone. These invading fibroblasts actually became small 'bioreactors' for formation of bone once the expression plasmid DNA was incorporated into their own genetic apparatus [Fang et al., 1996].

Finally, there is the possibility of directly incorporating cells derived from the marrow into a scaffold and transplanting it directly into the defect in vivo. Friedenstein et al. [1976] was the first to demonstrate the presence of a bone marrow-derived stromal cell population with osteogenic potential. These MSCs are strongly adherent to the substrate in tissue culture flasks and can be distinguished from hematopoietic cells and macrophages by a number of morphological, histochemical, and biochemical characteristics. Cultured bone marrow stromal cells (BMSCs) maintain many of the multipotential, differentiative features that define a stem cell; that is, they are capable of self-renewal and they can differentiate into several phenotypes including bone [Owen, 1988; Gundle et al., 1995]. Thus, in vitro expanded BMSCs may be a rich source of osteogenic progenitor cells that are capable of promoting the repair or regeneration of craniofacial osseous defects.

Several research groups have modified in vitro culture methods to expand marrow stromal cells derived from mouse and human bone marrow aspirates. They have successfully shown that these cells are capable of forming new bone in an in vivo animal model within a number of different vehicles [Owen, 1988; Gundle et al., 1995; Krebsbach et al., 1997, 1999; Kuznetsov et al., 1997]. Several factors may determine the success of this transplantation strategy including the species of cells transplanted, the surface chemistry of the scaffold material, the pore size of the scaffold, and the method of obtaining and culturing of the cells. To date, the most successful osteogenesis by transplanted human BMSCs has best been achieved on scaffolds that contain HA [Haynesworth, 1992; Krebsbach et al., 1997, 1999; Martin et al., 1997]. Several new bioresorbable materials are currently being developed and may be useful in the future for cell-based therapeutic approaches to craniofacial skeletal reconstruction.

In summary, the future for the use of a biomimetic approach in tissue engineering and TMJ reconstruction is encouraging. The advances in image-based design, solid free-form fabrication and stem cell biology may now make it possible to engineer patient-specific hybrid bone and cartilage constructs that could be used for TMJ or small joint (metacarpal and metatarsal) reconstruction. The ability to develop bone and cartilage constructs for joint repair may be possible in the not so distant future. Individuals have already initiated studies for development of the knee meniscus through the use of tissue-engineered constructs of collagen and glycosyaminoglycan matrices loaded with cells derived from the meniscus [Mueller et al., 1999] as well as small joints [Isogai et al., 1999].

References

Bell, E. (1995) Strategy for the selection of scaffolds for tissue engineering. Tissue Eng *1:* 163–179.

Brady, G.A., T.M. Chu, J.W. Halloran (1996) Curing behavior of ceramic resin for stereolithography; in Beaman, J.J., J.W. Barlow, D.L. Bourell, R.H. Crawford (eds): Solid Free Form Fabrication Proceedings. Solid Free Form Symposium, Austin, pp 403–410.

Brekke, J.H., J.M. Toth (1998) Principles of tissue engineering applied to programmable osteogenesis. J Biomed Mater Res (Apple Biomater) *43:* 380–398.

Bruder, S.P., K.H. Kraus, V.M. Goldberg, S. Kadiyala (1998) Critical-sized canine segmental femoral defects are healed by autologous mesenchymal stem cell therapy. 44th Ann Meet Orthop Res Soc, p 147.

Bruder, S.P., D.J. Fink, A.I. Caplan (1994) Mesenchymal stem cells in bone development, bone repair and skeletal regeneration therapy. J Cell Biochem *56:* 283–294.

Chu, T.M., J.W. Halloran (1997) Hydroxyapatite for implant fabrication by stereolithograph case studies of ceramic product development, manufacturing, and commercialization; in Ghosh, A., B. Hiremath, R. Barks (eds): Ceramic Transactions, vol 75. American Ceramics Society, Westerville.

Chu, T.M., J.W. Halloran, S.J. Hollister (1998) Hydroxyapatite scaffolds with controlled porosity. Ann Meet Am Ceramic Soc, May 3–6, 1998, Cincinnati.

Copray, J.C.V.M., H.W.B. Jansen, H.S. Duterloo (1985) The role of biomechanical factors in mandibular condylar cartilage growth and remodeling in vitro; in Carlson, D.S., J.A. McNamara, K. Ribbens (eds): Developmental Aspects of Temporomandibular Joint Disorders. Monograph Number 16: Craniofacial Growth Series. Ann Arbor, Center for Human Growth and Development, The University of Michigan, pp 235–269.

Dennis, J.E., S.E. Haynesworth, R.G. Young, A.I. Caplan (1992) Osteogenesis in marrow-derived mesenchymal cell porous ceramic composites transplanted subcutaneously: Effect of fibronectin and laminin on cell retention and rate of osteogenic expression. Cell Transplant *1:* 23–32.

Dunn, J.C.Y., R.G. Tompkins, M.L. Yarmush (1991) Long-term in vitro function of adult hepatocytes in a collagen sandwich configuration. Biotechnol Progr *7:* 237–245.

Fang, J., Y.Y. Zhu, E. Smiley, et al. (1996) Stimulation of new bone formation by direct transfer of osteogenic plasmid genes. Proc Natl Acad Sci USA *93:* 5753–5758.

Friedenstein, A.J., U.F. Gorskaja, N.N. Kulagina (1976) Fibroblast precursors in normal and irradiated mouse hematopoietic organs. Exp Hematol *4:* 267–274.

Gauthier, O., J.M. Bouler, E. Aguado, et al. (1998) Macroporous biphasic calcium phosphate ceramics: Influence of macropore diameter and macroporosity percentage on bone ingrowth. Biomaterials *19:* 133–139.

Griffith, M.L., T.M. Chu, W. Wagner, J.W. Halloran (1995) Ceramic stereolithography for investment casting and biomedical applications; in Marcus, H.L., J.J. Beaman, J.W. Barlow, D.L. Bourell, R.H. Crawford (eds): Solid Free Form Fabrication Proceedings, Solid Free Form Symposium, Austin.

Guldberg, R. (1997) Pers. commun.

Gundle, R., C.J. Joyner, J.T. Triffitt (1995) Human bone tissue formation in diffusion chamber culture in vivo by bone-derived cells and marrow stromal fibroblastic cells. Bone *16:* 597–601.

Haynesworth, S.E., J. Goshima, V.M. Goldberg, A.I. Caplan (1992) Characterization of cells with osteogenic potential from human marrow. Bone *13:* 81–88.

Hollister, S.J., R. Levy, T.M. Chu, et al. (1997) Design and manufacture of a porous orbital floor scaffold using image processing and rapid prototyping. Proc ASME Summer Meet.

Hollister, S.J., T.M. Chu, R. Guldberg, et al. (1998) Design and manufacture of HA biomaterial scaffolds for bone tissue engineering. 44th Ann Meet Orthop Res Soc, p 423.

Hollister, S.J, J.W. Halloran, T.M. Chu, et al. (2000) An image-based approach for designing and manufacturing craniofacial scaffolds. Int J Oral Maxillofac Surg *29:* 67–71.

Ingber, D. (1993) The riddle of morphogenesis: A question of solution chemistry or molecular engineering? Cell *75:* 1249–1252.

Isogai, N., W. Landis, et al. (1999) Formation of phalanges and small joints by tissue-engineering. J Bone Joint Surg *81(A):* 306–316.

Iwasaki, M., K. Nakata, H. Nakahara, et al. (1993) Transforming growth factor-β1 stimulates chondrogenesis and inhibits osteogenesis in high density culture of periosteum-derived cells. Endocrinology *132:* 1603–1608.

Iwasaki, M., H. Nakahara, K. Nakata, et al. (1995) Regulation of proliferation and osteochondrogenic differentiation of periosteum-derived cells by transforming growth factor-β and basic fibroblast growth factor. J Bone Joint Surg *77-A:* 543–554.

Izumi, T., S.P. Scully, A. Heydemann, et al. (1992) Transforming growth factor β1 stimulates type II collagen expression in cultured periosteum-derived cells. J Bone Miner Res *7:* 115–121.

Jacobs, P. (1992) Stereolithography and RP & M Technologies. ASME, Dearborn.

Jin, Q.-M., H. Takita, T. Kohgo, K. Atsumi, H. Itoh, Y. Kuboki (2000) Effects of geometry of hydroxyapatite as a cell substratum in BMP-induced ectopic bone formation. J Biomed Mater Res *51:* 491–499.

Kadiyala, S., N. Jaiswal, S.P. Bruder (1997) Culture-expanded, bone marrow-derived mesenchymal stem cells can regenerate a critical-sized segmental bone defect. Tissue Eng *3:* 173–185.

Krebsbach, P.H., S.A. Kuznetsov, K. Satomura, et al. (1997) Bone formation in vivo: Comparison of osteogenesis by transplanted mouse and human marrow stromal fibroblasts. Transplantation *63:* 1059–1069.

Krebsbach, P.H., S.A. Kuznetsov, P. Bianco, et al. (1999) Bone marrow stromal cells: Characterization and clinical application. Crit Rev Oral Biol Med *10:* 165–181.

Kuboki, Y., T. Saito, M. Murata, et al. (1995) Two distinctive BMP-carriers induce zonal chondrogenesis and membraneous ossification, respectively; geometrical factors of matrices for cell differentiation. Connect Tiss Res *32:* 219–226.

Kühne, J.H., R. Bartl, B. Frisch, et al. (1994) Bone formation in coralline hydroxyapatite: Effects of pore size studied in rabbits. Acta Orthop Scand *65:* 246–252.

Kuznetsov, S.A., P.H. Krebsbach, K. Satomura, et al. (1997) Single-colony derived strains of human stromal fibroblasts form bone after transplantation in vivo. J Bone Miner Res *12:* 1335–1347.

Langer, R., J.P. Vacanti (1993) Tissue engineering. Science *260:* 920–926.

Levy, R.A., T.M. Chu, J.W. Halloran, et al. (1997) CT-generated porous hydroxyapatite floor prosthesis as a prototype bioimplant. Am J Neuroradiol *18:* 1522–1525.

Martin, I., A. Muraglia, G. Campanile, et al. (1997) Fibroblastic growth factor-2 supports 'ex vivo' expansion and maintenance of osteogenic precursors from human bone marrow. Endocrinology *138:* 4456–4462.

Meikle, M.C. (1992) Remodeling; in Sarnat, B.G., D.M. Laskin (eds): The Temporomandibular Joint: A Biological Basis for Clinical Practice, ed 4. Philadelphia, Saunders, pp 93–107.

Mercuri, L.G. (1998) Alloplastic temporomandibular joint reconstruction. Oral Surg Oral Med Oral Pathol *85:* 631–637.

Mueller, S.M., S. Shortfroff, T.O. Schneider, et al. (1999) Meniscus cells seeded in type I and type II collagen-GAG matrices in vitro. Biomaterials *20:* 701–709.

Nehrer, S., H.A. Breinan, A. Ramappa, et al. (1997) Matrix collagen type and pore size influence behaviour of seeded canine chondrocytes. Biomaterials *18:* 769–776.

Owen, M. (1988) Marrow stromal stem cells. J Cell Sci *10 (suppl):* 63–76.

Perrott, D.H., H. Umeda, L.B. Kaban (1994) Costochondral graft reconstruction: Reconstruction of the ramus/condyle unit: Long term follow-up. Int J Oral Maxillofac Surg *23:* 321–328.

Raustia, A., H. Pernu, J. Pyhtinen, et al. (1996) Clinical and computed tomographic findings in costochondral grafts replacing the mandibular condyle. J Oral Maxillofac Surg *54:* 1393–1400.

Ripamonti, U., S. Ma, A.H. Reddi (1992) The critical role of geometry of porous hydroxyapatite delivery system in induction of bone by osteogenin, a bone morphologenetic protein. Matrix *12:* 202–212.

Rubin, J.P., M.J. Yaremchuk (1997) Complications and toxicities of implantable biomaterials used in facial reconstructive and aesthetic surgery: A comprehensive review of the literature. Plast Rec Surg *100:* 1336–1353.

Sampson, D., et al. (1999) Pers. commun., www.tmjconcepts.com.

Shi, S., M. Kirk, A. Kahn (1996) The role of type I collagen in the regulation of the osteoblast phenotype. J Bone Miner Res *11:* 1139–1145.

Tsuruga, E., H. Takita, H. Itoh, et al. (1997) Pore size of porous hydroxyapatite as the cell-substratum controls BMP-induced osteogenesis. J Biochem *121:* 317–324.

Van Loon, J.P., L.G.M. De Bont, G. Boering (1995) Evaluation of temporomandibular joint prosthesis: Review of the literature from 1946 to 1994 and implications for future prosthesis designs. J Oral Maxillofac Surg *53:* 984–996.

Zysset, P.K., A.L. Marsan, T.M. Chu, et al. (1997) Rapid prototyping of trabecular bone for mechanical testing. Proc ASME Summer Bioengineering Meet.

Author Index Vol. 169, No. 3, 2001

Cells Tissues Organs

Subject Index Vol. 169, No. 3, 2001

KARGER

Fax +41 61 306 12 34
E-Mail karger@karger.ch
www.karger.com

Accessible online at:
www.karger.com/journals/cto

Cells
Tissues
Organs

Conference Calendar

July 2001 **Madrid** Spain	10th Congress of European Federation of Biotechnology	**Information:** DECHEMA, Theodor-Heuss-Allee 25, D–60061 Frankfurt/M, Germany Fax +49 69 7564 201, E-Mail info@dechema.de
1.7.–6.7.2001 **Singapore**	International Conference on Materials for Advanced Technologies (ICMAT 2001) Singapore International Conventiom and Exhibition Center Organised by: Materials Research Society	**Information:** Conference Secretariat, AV Consultants Pte Ltd, 232-A River Valley Road, Singapore 238290 Tel. (65) 735 625, Fax (65) 735 2091, E-Mail icmat2001@pacific.net.sg, http://www.mrs.org.sg/icmat2001
4.7.–6.7.2001 **Aachen** Germany	5th International Conference on Cellular Engineering	**Information:** Christina Kellemen, Univ. Appl. Sci. Aachen, Ginsterweg 1, D–52428 Juelich Tel. +49 2461 993244, Fax: +49 2461 993199
8.7.–12.7.2001 **Kyoto** Japan	14th International Congress of Developmental Biology	**Information:** Secretariat of 14th ICDB, c/o Congress Corporation, Kinki Invention Center Bldg., 14 Yoshida Kawahara-cho, Sakyo-ku, Kyoto 606-8305 (Japan) Tel. +81 75 752 0888, Fax +81 75 762 2304, E-Mail isdb@congre.co.jp, http://www.congre.co.jp/icdb/
11.7.–13.7.2001 **Dublin** Ireland	Anatomical Society of Great Britain and Ireland Summer Meeting on 'The Respiratory System'	**Information:** Dr. Jonathan P. Bennett, Division of Biomedical Science, Imperial College of Medicine, St. Mary's Campus, South Kensington, GB–London SW7 2AZ Tel. +44 (0)171 594 31 66, Fax +44 (0)171 594 31 69, E-Mail J.p.bennett@ic.ac.uk
18.7.–22.7.2001 **Seattle, Wash.** USA	Society for Developmental Biology 60th Annual Meeting	**Information:** SDB, 9650 Rockville Pike, Bethesda, MD 20814-3998, USA http://www.sdbonline.org
22.7.–26.7.2001 **Sun City** South Africa	XVth International Symposium on Morphological Sciences	**Information:** Professor H.B. Groenewald, University of Pretoria, Scientific Secretariat, XVIth ISMS, Department of Anatomy, Faculty of Veterinary Science, Private Bag X04, Onderstepoort 0110 (Republic of South Africa) Tel. +27 12 529 8247, Fax +27 12 529 8320, E-Mail hgroenew@opup.ac.za, http://www.satic.co.za/assa
4.9.–5.9.2001 **Hartshill** UK	Cell and Tissue Engineering Society 3rd Annual Meeting	**Information:** Prof. Alicia El Haj, Centre for Science and Technology in Medicine, Keele University, Hartshill, ST4 7QB, UK, Tel. 00 44 1782 554253, E-Mail a.j.el.haj@keele.ac.uk, http://www.keele.ac.uk/depts/stm/cellular/ctes_2.htm
9.9.–14.9.2001 **Rome** Italy	14th World Congress of Union Internationale de Phlébologie	**Information:** GC Congressi, Via P. Borsieri, 12, I–00185 Roma (Italy) Tel. +39 06 370 0541, Fax +39 06 373 52337, E-Mail angiolsg@pronet.it
20.9.–22.9.2001 **Greifswald** Germany	11. Teratologie-Symposium Methoden der experimentellen Teratologie, Klinische Teratologie	**Information:** Prof. Dr. med. Jochen Fanghänel, Universität Greifswald, Institut für Anatomie, Friedrich-Loefller-Strasse 23c, D–17487 Greifswald Tel. +49 (0)3834 86 53 00, Fax +49 (0)3834 86 53 02, E-Mail fanghaen@rz.uni-greifswald.de

KARGER
Fax + 41 61 306 12 34
E-Mail karger@karger.ch
www.karger.com

Accessible online at:
www.karger.com/journals/cto

26.9–28.9.2001 **Würzburg** Germany	18. Arbeitstagung der Anatomischen Gesellschaft	**Information:** Anatomisches Institut, Koellikerstrasse 6, Würzburg Tel. +49 931 31 27 03
30.9.–3.10.2001 **Granada** Spain	43rd International Meeting of the European Tissue Culture Society Cell Interactions and Cellular Complexity	**Information:** ETCS 2001 Meeting, Unidad de Hepatología Experimental, Centro de Investigación, Hospital La Fe, Avda. Campanar, 21, E–46009 Valencia (Spain) E-Mail etcs_esp@gva.es, http://www.san.gva.es/centros/lafe/ETCS/ ETCS_ESP-granada-2001-00.html
October 2001 **Algarve** Portugal	Course in: Polymer Based Systems in Tissue Engineering, Replacement and Regeneration	**Information:** Rui L. Reis, Dept. Polymer Eng., Univ. Minho, Campus de Gualtar, P–4710-057 Braga, Portugal E-Mail rgreis@eng.uminho.pt
9.10.–10.10.2001 **Hannover** Germany	International Conference in the Field of Tissue Engineering Second Transdisciplinary Conference on Principles and Perspectives in Regenerative Medicine	**Information:** Congress Secretariat, NATI Technologieagentur Niedersachsen GmbH, Heike Ewering, Wahrenwalder Str. 7, D–30165 Hannover Tel. +49 5 11 93 57 1 20, Fax +49 5 11 93 57 4 39, E-Mail regmed@nati.de
7.11.–9.11.2001 **Strasbourg** France	Société de Biologie Cellulaire de France Deutsche Gesellschaft für Zellbiologie e.V. First Joint French-German Congress on Cell Biology	**Information:** Deutsche Gesellschaft für Zellbiologie e.V., Deutsches Krebsforschungszentrum, Im Neuenheimer Feld 280, D–69120 Heidelberg Tel. +49 6221 42 3451, Fax +49 6221 42 3452, E-Mail DGZ@DKFZ-Heidelberg.de
7.11.–10.11.2001 **Freiburg i.Br.** Germany	First Biennial Meeting of the European Tissue Engineering Society (ETES)	**Information:** Ms. Andrea Kricheldorf, k + k Kongress und Kommunikation, Hugstetter Strasse 55, D–79106 Freiburg (Germany) Tel. +49 761 270 7316, Fax +49 761 270 7317, E-Mail kkkri@sun11.ukl.uni-freiburg.de
June 2002 **Seoul** South Korea	29th International Symposium on Controlled Release of Bioactive Materials	**Information:** Controlled Release Society Inc., 1020 Milwaukee Ave, Suite 335, Deerfield, IL 60015, USA Fax +1 847 808 7073, E-Mail crs@crsadmndq.org
July 2002 **Seattle, Wash.** USA	53rd Annual Meeting of the Histochemical Society	**Information:** HS, Univ. Washington, Neurology Dept., UW Box 356465, Seattle, WA 98195, USA Fax +1 206 764 2164, E-Mail wistahl@u.washington.edu
14.7.–19.7.2002 **Florence** Italy	6th International Conference Materials in Clinical Applications	**Information:** CIMTEC 2002 Secretariat, P.O. Box 174, I–48018 Faenza, Italy Tel. +39 0546 22461/664143, Fax +39 0546 664138/663362 or visit CIMTEC 2002 web site: www.dinamica.it/cimtec
11.9.–15.9.2002 **Timişoara** Romania	XVIIth International Symposium on Morphological Sciences	**Information:** Prof. Dr. med. Petru Matusz, Scientific Secretariat, Department of Anatomy, University of Medicine and Pharmacy 'Victor Babes', Piata Eftimie Murgu 2, RO–1900 Timişoara Fax +40 56 190 626, E-Mail matusz@umft.ro, Website: www.isms.2002.dnttm.ro
14.12.–18.12.2002 **San Francisco, Calif.** USA	42nd Annual Convent of the American Society for Cell Biology	**Information:** ASCB, 9650 Rockville Pike, Bethesda, MD 20814, USA Fax +1 301 530 7139, E-Mail enewman@ascb.org